P9-CBX-914

Dedicated to all seekers of better health who believe
in the natural approach.

Published by Maps Publishing
P.O. Box 681264
San Antonio, Texas 78268

First Printing – 5,000
May, 1988

Second Printing – 5,000
March, 1989

Maps Publishing does not directly or indirectly dispense medical
advise or prescribe the use of herbs, vitamins, minerals, etc., as a form
of treatment for sickness without medical approval.

The purpose and beauty of this work is in the fact that it provides you with both the way to determine what your nutritional needs may be and how to satisfy those needs.

This booklet contains a questionnaire that is suitable for every member of your family. Once the questions are answered you simply use the answer page to determine what the solutions are for the particular problems discussed.

Each answer provides you with a synergistically complete nutritional support program, that may be available in the health food store today. In addition to supplement suggestions there are foods, drinks and other beneficial knowledge provided.

This is the kind of book that should be in every household because of its thoroughness in dealing with and treating the most common ailments that families face in today's world.

TABLE OF CONTENTS

Preface

Every health book on the shelves today is the result of someone's desire to help others. Some of the books are written by research people, medical practitioners, and others with particular philosophies. Hardly any are written by practicing NATUROPATHS.

A NATUROPATH is someone who follows the "PATH OF NATURE" in the course of healing.

As a NATUROPATH who has been practicing the healing art since 1973 I have come to learn a lot about NATURAL HEALING. I have come to understand that not everything that is written by the researcher works. Therefore you must experiment to find what truly works.

Even within the experimentation you learn that 90% of what you do will help 90% of the people 90% of the time. There is always the 10% that will not benefit. The reasons for this are many, some are nutritional imbalances brought on by medications that are so bad that it would take years to correct the situation, others, the psychological aspects would work against healing. And there are other reasons.

The purpose of this book is to present to you programs that are both NATUROPATHIC in design as well as SYNERGISTIC in effect. I learned through my many years of counselling that when you combine herbs with vitamins or minerals and other nutrients you get a far superior nutritional support program. This is essentially the SYNERGISTIC effect.

It is my desire and "calling" to bring this information to you. To provide you with nutritional programs that are effective, easy to work with and inexpensive to purchase.

I personally guarantee you that if you work with my SYNERGISTIC NATUROPATHIC SUPPORT PROGRAMS you will benefit immensely.

GOOD HEALTH,

NEIL KELLY

Introduction _____

For every effect in life there is a cause. There is not one instance where this truth is violated. However there are many different causes, or so it appears.

The only way to determine the cause is through investigative work. And you must work backwards in order to arrive at the true starting point. This is what medical and nutritional sciences try to do. There are disagreements between the two branches of science on some levels, but not all.

In fact there are many diseases that are the result of nutritional deficiencies that the medical community recognizes but does not necessarily admit.

Our purpose here is to 'backtrack' to those nutritional causes of the most common disease and how to refortify the body with the correct nutrients that will stop the disease from progressing. Through the administration of the proper nutrients it may also become very possible and highly likely that the body will be put into a healing mode. It is known, and would be readily admitted to by an aware doctor, that the body heals itself. All that the drugs do is to deal with the symptoms while your body goes through the healing cycle. Of course this assumes that your problem is viral/germ oriented. If, on the other hand, your condition is of "unknown" causes then the prescriptions are there to control the symptoms. NOT TO DEAL WITH THE CAUSE.

This booklet will provide you with knowledge and with the "know how" of what to do to heal yourself where possible. In those instances where you are dealing with a problem that has no "known" cause, then you will have the information that you need to exercise control over the problem. Who knows, by exercising control and placing yourself on a sound nutritional program you just may bring about a "cure" to another "unknown" caused disease.

It is our intent to give to you complete nutritional programs that will help you to improve your condition, regardless of what it may be.

For each condition you will find nutritional as well as dietary suggestions. In addition to these you will also find, when appropriate, the exercises or drinks or other therapies that will be beneficial. Like everything in life, for something to work it must be employed properly and with continuity. With these words we will begin our journey toward a new and more vibrant picture of health.

Nutritional Supplements As Healers

Even though the role of nutritional supplements as a healing modality is recognized and accepted by most health conscious consumers, many find themselves hampered by a lack of basic knowledge when it comes to creating a nutritional support program for themselves. Some consumers find current approaches to nutritional support programs complicated and not as effective as they would like, while others find nutritional programs difficult to work with. Some people find them time consuming and costly.

The purpose of this Guide Book is to overcome those roadblocks and make nutritional support an effective, affordable and workable part of every consumer's desire to heal themselves. To accomplish this, NEIL KELLY has developed comprehensive synergistically complete naturopathic support programs to meet the needs of most. Each naturopathic program is complete with the vitamins, minerals, herbs and additional nutrients essential to lasting results. All the naturopathic programs offered are based on years of actual clinical experience and are guaranteed effective. By following the steps outlined in this guide book, nutritional needs can be identified in a matter of minutes. And a synergistically complete program can be created quickly and inexpensively.

Synergism

Synergism is defined as "The mutually cooperating action of separate substances which together produce an effect greater than that of any component taken alone"(Funk & Wagnalls New International Dictionary).

Now when you take that definition and apply it to a nutritional formula you can begin to imagine the benefits. First, you have the convenience of taking fewer tablets to accomplish your healing goals. Second, you potentiate that which you are doing so that each individual property of the herb, vitamin or other nutrient is magnified. This process of magnification gives you a quicker healing response and a more complete one when you take the correct formula for your condition.

Determining
Nutritional Needs _____

Therapeutic nutritional needs are simply a reflection of symptoms and conditions that are directly related to the affect of nutritional deficits on the various body systems. When the supply of nutrients in the foods we eat do not keep up with the demand of today's environment and lifestyles, the result is a nutritional deficit.

Nutritional deficits manifest themselves in a variety of ways. For some people the affect is a weakened musculo-skeletal system that may appear as various aches and pains or contribute to the malfunction of other body systems. For other people, the affect may be on the immune system. They find themselves in a continuous run down state and are often subject to colds, flu and viruses. Some people manifest cardiovascular symptoms such as high blood pressure or poor circulation. Another affect may involve blood sugar regulation in the form of hypoglycemia or diabetes. The list goes on in the ways that nutritional deficits affect body systems.

Each body system is dependent on specific nutrients for proper function. By linking conditions and specific combinations of symptoms, it is possible to identify appropriate nutritional support needed to overcome nutritional deficits. Using this concept, NEIL KELLY has developed naturopathic support programs for common conditions and illnesses.

The Condition/Symptom Survey Form, shown on page 7, is the vehicle used to link conditions and symptoms to the appropriate nutrition support program. Simply check the conditions and symptoms that apply to you. By using the Key, shown on page 9, you can quickly identify the naturopathic support program that will support the appropriate body systems.

Support Program Conversion Key

1. The Condition / Symptom Form and Conversion Key are divided into seven groups. Groups 2 through 8 divide common symptoms and conditions by body systems.

Group 2	=	neuro-endocrine
Group 3	=	musculoskeletal
Group 4	=	immune
Group 5	=	skin
Group 6	=	cardiovascular
Group 7	=	reproductive
Group 8	=	muscles
Group 9	=	miscellaneous

Group One correlates various symptoms with a variety of body systems and relates specifically to CANDIDA ALBICANS.

2. Align the number on the support Programs Conversion Key with the Conditions / Symptoms Survey Form.

3. Record all X's next to corresponding numbers on the Support Programs Conversion Key.

4. To determine if a nutritional support program is indicated in Group One, total the X's in Group One and add them to the total number of X's in Group Seven. If there are seven or more X's, the symptoms are almost certainly yeast connected.

When you suspect a yeast connection, the nutritional support program for candida and a yeast control diet is indicated. If number 45 in Group Seven is marked with an X and a yeast connection is suspected, the formula for douching should be used as an additional support program.

NOTE: See pages 9 and 10 for foods that you can and can't eat on a yeast control diet.

5. In Groups 2 through 8, each X indicates a nutritional support program designed to support body systems associated with specific symptoms or conditions.

Determining Priorities

1. The number one priority in providing nutritional support is to build on a solid foundation. NEIL KELLY has developed a unique two phase foundation to meet the nutritional need of every person seeking to have a complete program. For males, Formula M-M, or, Formula M-W, for females. These nutritional support programs are designed to be taken in the mornings.

Formula M-M/H, a multi-mineral should be taken at bed time. Every person on a specific nutritional support program should have Formula M-M or Formula M-F plus Formula M-M/H as the foundation of their nutritional regimen.

2. If a nutritional support program is indicated in Group One, it takes priority over nutritional support programs indicated in any other Group.

3. When there are multiple X's in Groups 2 through 8, priorities must be set.

    a. Identify the most acute conditions or symptoms to work with first.

    b. Avoid using more than two nutritional support programs (in addition to the basic foundation formulas) at any one time.

    c. At the end of one month, reevaluate your progress with the Condition/Symptom Survey and begin nutritional support of chronic conditions and symptoms where indicated.

Self Therapy Questionnaire _____

Please read instructions before completing this questionnaire.

INSTRUCTIONS FOR USING THE CONDITION/SYMPTOM SURVEY FORM

Place an X on the line next to the conditions which apply to you. Only place an X next to those symptoms or conditions that are current; not something that happened three months or a year ago.

Any condition that is controlled by medication is considered current. Example: If you have high blood pressure and it is normal while on medication, you should still place an X on the line next to high blood pressure.

Be sure to respond to all eight groups.

GROUP ONE

1. _____ Crave sugar, bread or alcoholic beverages?
2. _____ Recurrent digestive symptoms?
4. _____ Suffer from hives, psoriasis or other skin rashes?
5. _____ Are you bothered by fatigue, depression or poor memory?
6. _____ Have you taken repeated rounds of antibiotics?
7. _____ Are you bothered by headaches, muscle and joint pains or incoordination?
8. _____ Does exposure to tobacco, perfume or other chemical odors provoke moderate to sever symptoms?
9. _____ Do you suffer from alternating diarrhea/constipation?
10. _____ Do you feel bad all over with no diagnosed cause?

GROUP TWO

11. _____ Diabetic tendencies? (excessive thirst, frequent urination, increased appetite, and loss of weight.)
12. _____ Mood swings?
13. _____ Low blood sugar? (wake up tired, no energy in afternoon, sleepy after meals, and get upset easily.)
13. _____ Excess anxiety?
14. _____ Tension headaches?
15. _____ Low energy level?
16. _____ Exhaustion following stressful situations?

GROUP THREE

17. _____ Arthritic tendencies?
18. _____ Female over 50?
19. _____ Osteoporosis?
20. _____ Musculoskeletal injury?
21. _____ Arthritic joint pains?
22. _____ Musculoskeletal aches?

GROUP FOUR

23. _____ Frequent colds or flu?
24. _____ Frequent allergies?
25. _____ Stuffy nose?
26. _____ Respiratory congestion?
27. _____ Sinus headaches?
28. _____ Ear infections?

GROUP FIVE

29. _____ Psoriasis?
30. _____ Warts?
31. _____ Itchy skin rash?
32. _____ Fungus on skin or nails?
33. _____ Acne?
34. _____ Skin irritation?
35. _____ Hemorrhoidal itch?

GROUP SIX

36. _____ High blood pressure?
37. _____ High cholesterol?
38. _____ Poor circulation? (cold hands, feet, numbness in toes, fingers, slight loss of hearing, excessive hair loss, and dizziness when standing quickly.)
39. _____ Fluid retention?
40. _____ Overweight?

GROUP SEVEN

Male

41. _____ Prostatitis?
42. _____ Loss of sexual interest?
43. _____ Infertility?
44. _____ Impotence?

Female

45. _____ Vaginitis?
46. _____ Loss of sexual interest?
47. _____ Menstrual difficulties?
48. _____ Premenstrual tension?
49. _____ Have you taken birth control pills?

GROUP EIGHT

50. _____ Backaches?
51. _____ Leg aches?
52. _____ Difficult time falling asleep?
53. _____ Toe cramps, "charlie horses"?

GROUP NINE

54. _____ Do you have ulcers?
55. _____ Do you have frequent loss of memory?
56. _____ Do you have Alzheimer's?
57. _____ Do you have cataracts or glaucoma?
58. _____ Do you have asthma?
59. _____ Do you have emphysema?
60. _____ Do you have gall stones?
61. _____ Do you have kidney stones?

Support Program Conversion Key _____

The following letter abbreviations, such as M-DER, refer to programs listed in the directory.

GROUP ONE

1-9. This section correlates candidiasis symptoms and should combine with responses from Group Seven. If there are one or more checks the symptoms are almost certainly yeast connected. When you suspect a yeast connection, nutritional support Formula M-C/A and a yeast control diet is indicated.

GROUP TWO

10. _____ PAGE 41
11. _____ PAGE 55
12. _____ PAGE 55
13. _____ PAGE 41, 86
14. _____ PAGE 41, 86, 100
15. _____ PAGE 55
16. _____ PAGE 55

GROUP THREE

17. _____ PAGE 23
18. _____ PAGE 76
19. _____ PAGE 76
20. _____ PAGE 7
21. _____ PAGE 100
22. _____ PAGE 100

GROUP FOUR

23. _____ PAGE 38
24. _____ PAGE 21
25. _____ PAGE 40, 101
26. _____ PAGE 40, 99
27. _____ PAGE 100
28. _____ PAGE 99

GROUP FIVE

29. _____ PAGE 19, 100
30. _____ PAGE 19, 100
31. _____ PAGE 19, 101
32. _____ PAGE 19, 97
33. _____ PAGE 19, 97
34. _____ PAGE 19, 97
35. _____ PAGE 99

GROUP SIX

36. _____ PAGE 53
37. _____ PAGE 35
38. _____ PAGE 35
39. _____ PAGE 93
40. _____ PAGE 61, 93

NOTE: Each person should be on a nutritional foundation program such as M-M (Male) or M-W (Female) along with M-M/H.

GROUP SEVEN

Male
41. _____ PAGE 84
42. _____ PAGE 45
43. _____ PAGE 45
44. _____ PAGE 61

Female
45. _____ PAGE 101
46. _____ PAGE 45
47. _____ PAGE 45
48. _____ PAGE 45
49. _____ Correlate with Group One.

GROUP EIGHT

50. _____ PAGE 14
51. _____ PAGE 14
52. _____ PAGE 14, 86
53. _____ PAGE 14

GROUP NINE

54. _____ PAGE 91
55. _____ PAGE 70
56. _____ PAGE 70
57. _____ PAGE 31, 49
58. _____ PAGE 8, 40
59. _____ PAGE 45, 40
60. _____ PAGE 48
61. _____ PAGE 66, 65

Nutritional Support
Program Instructions

The following pages list instructions for each synergistically complete nutritional support program.

The purpose of the program instruction information is to simplify the therapeutic use of each nutritional support program.

Once the correct program is identified, it becomes necessary to work with the most effective "usage suggestions" to gain the quickest results. Herein lies the value of the following information. Instructions for each nutritional support program indicate exactly how many tablets and how frequently they should be taken, depending upon whether or not the condition or symptoms are acute or chronic. Also included in the instructions are those additional factors (foods, beverages, exercise, etc.) to be used or avoided.

Synergistically
Complete Programs

Those of us involved in the art of natural healing and health are very well aware of the need for certain nutrients at special times in specific amounts. Every time we form a nutritional program for someone we draw on that knowledge and understanding, (certain nutrients in specific amounts at special times).

The clear-cut examples of this truth are demonstrated in the varying amounts of zinc, calcium, B-complex, pantothenic acid and the lipo-tropic vitamins that are needed at the different age levels of growing children and adults.

Children require extra amounts of zinc and calcium during the pre-teen years to strengthen the growth of bones as well as the reproductive system.

During the teen years additional choline and inositol would be wise to bring into the nutritional program to offset the accumulation of fats that have been generated by the "burger and french fry" diet.

Zinc during this time period is also important because of its role in skin care and the role it plays in the development of anti-bodies in the immune system. Pantothenic acid should also be increased to help the teenager in dealing with the competitive stress of growing up and dealing with life.

Stress continues to mount as we grow into adulthood and so our requirements for additional pantothenic acid, calcium, B12, iron and zinc is also increased. During this same period of time an increase in the lipotropic vitamins (fat burners) is also highly advisable because of the elevated amounts of cholesterol and triglycerides found in the blood stream of most adults.

With these understandings the following nutritional support programs were created.

Directory of Synergistically Complete Naturopathic Programs

Nutritional Foundation
For Everybody

PROGRAM M-M/H

Should be a Multi-Mineral and Herb combination that is designed for the entire family. This type of formulation is part of the foundation for all nutritional support programs.

It should also contain those herbs that will ensure the highest rate of assimilation.

Here are the prime nutrients that would be beneficial:

Calcium (Amino Acid Chelate)
GTF Chromium
Iodine (Kelp)
Iron (Amino Acid Chelate)
Magnesium (Amino Acid Chelate)
Manganese (Amino Acid Chelate)
Phosphorus (Amino Acid Chelate)
Potassium (Amino Acid Complex)
Selenium (Amino Acid Chelate)
Zinc (Amino Acid Chelate)
Pumpkin Seeds
Alfalfa
Yellow Dock
Beets
Chaparral
Red Clover
Marshmallow Root
Horsetail Grass

HERBS to provide synergistic compliment.

Knowing that you can find these nutrients in a formula that will deliver most of the prime ingredients, here is how I recommend to take them: 3 at bedtime.

Nutritional Foundation
For Men

Should be a Multi-Vitamin and Herb combination that is especially designed for men (20 to 60). This type of formulation can be the foundation for all nutritional support programs.

Here is a formula that is available in the marketplace today that would be beneficial for providing most of the nutritional support for this condition:

VITAMIN A (Fish Liver Oil)
VITAMIN D (Fish Liver Oil)
VITAMIN E (D-Alpha Tocopherol)
VITAMIN F (Unsaturated Fatty Acids)
VITAMIN B1 (Thiamine)
VITAMIN B2 (Riboflavin)
VITAMIN B6 (Pyridoxine)
VITAMIN B12 (Cobalamin)
BIOTIN (vitamin H)
CHOLINE (choline bitartrate)
INOSITOL
FOLIC ACID (Folacin)
NIACINAMIDE
PANTOTHENIC ACID (B5)
PABA (Para Aminobenzoic Acid)
VITAMIN C (Ascorbic Acid)
BIOFLAVONOIDS (Vitamin P)
RUTIN
HESPERIDIN
IODINE (Kelp)
GINSENG
DAMIANA
SAW PALMETTO
SARSAPARILLA
DANDELION ROOT
LICORICE ROOT
PUMPKIN SEED
PARSLEY
BETAINE HCL

Here are the nutrients and why they help:

HERBS

HERBS that are specific to the male for extra synergistic benefits.
SIBERIAN GINSENG: Has been used for centuries as a tonic and is highly invigorating. It is also famous for "aphrodisiac" type properties. Beneficial in restoring mental abilities.
LICORICE: Nourishes the adrenal glands. Adjusts concentration of vital blood salts, thereby stimulating and sustaining proper adrenal function. Stimulates production of interferon.

DAMIANA: Beneficial on reproductive organs. Acts as a general tonic on nervous system.

SAW PALMETTO: Builds strength in testes and mammae. Valuable in all diseases of the reproductive organs (male and female). Helps restore function and nutritional support to all bodily systems.

SARSAPARILLA: Attacks microbial substances in the blood stream, neutralizing them.

DANDELION: Improves function of liver. Bile and certain enzymes produced in the liver aid in maintaining proper intestinal flora. Excellent for liver and kidneys. Purifies blood, destroys acids in blood.

PARSLEY: Known to reduce inflammation. Rich in Potassium. Diuretic. Invigorates the body. High in Vitamin A, C, and Provitamin A.

PUMPKIN SEEDS: High in zinc.

FALSE UNICORN: To strengthen fertility factors.

High points of this type of formulation would be additional:

PANTOTHENIC ACID: To fortify the body in dealing with stress.

CHOLINE/INOSITOL: For cholesterol reduction.

NIACINAMIDE: For opening arteries and allowing more blood to flow to vital organs and extremities (toes, fingers, eyes, and scalp).

Knowing that you can find these nutrients in a formula that will deliver most of the prime ingredients, here is how I recommend to take them: 2 at breakfast.

Nutritional Foundation
For Women

PROGRAM M-W

Should be a Multi-Vitamin and Herb combination that is especially designed for females (20 to 60). This type of formulation can be the foundation for all nutritional support programs.

Here is a formula that is available in the marketplace today that would be beneficial for providing most of the nutritional support for this condition:

VITAMIN A (Fish Liver Oil)
VITAMIN D (Fish Liver Oil)
VITAMIN E (D-Alpha Tocopherol)
VITAMIN F (Unsaturated Fatty Acids)
VITAMIN B1 (Thiamine)
VITAMIN B2 (Riboflavin)
VITAMIN B6 (Pyridoxine)
VITAMIN B12 (Cobalamin)
BIOTIN (Vitamin H)
CHOLINE (Choline Bitartrate)
INOSITOL
FOLIC ACID (Folacin)
NIACINAMIDE
PANTOTHENIC ACID
PABA (Para Aminobenzoic Acid)
VITAMIN C (Ascorbic Acid)
BIOFLAVONOIDS (Vitamin P)
RUTIN
HESPERIDIN
IODINE (Kelp)
BETAINE HCL
BLESSED THISTLE
FALSE UNICORN
LICORICE ROOT
WILD YAM ROOT
RED RASPBERRY
SQUAW VINE
DONG QUAI
DANDELION ROOT

Here are the nutrients and why they help:

HERBS

HERBS that are specific to the female for extra synergistic benefits.
ECHINACEA: Cleanses lymph system and improves antibody production. Blood purifier, lymphatic cleanser. Increases activity of white blood cells to be able to fight, destroy and eat toxic organisms.

DANDELION: Improves function of liver. Bile and certain enzymes produced in the liver aid in maintaining proper intestinal flora. Excellent for liver and kidneys. Purifies blood, destroys acids in blood, has beneficial effect on the female organs.

LICORICE ROOT and WILD YAM ROOT: These herbs have estrogen producing characteristics. Adjusts concentration of vital blood salts, thereby stimulating and sustaining proper adrenal function. Stimulates production of interferon. Estrogenic activity; a uterine tonic. Relaxing and soothing to the nerves. Excellent in glandular balance.

FALSE UNICORN: Known to strengthen female uterine walls. Cleanse and strengthen ovaries.

TANGKUEI *also known as* **DONG QUAI:** Is considered one of the best herbs for females because it does so many different things within the reproduction system. Excellent for all female conditions.

PARSLEY: Known to reduce inflammation. Rich in potassium, diuretic. Invigorates the body. High in Vitamin B, C and Provitamin A.

YELLOW DOCK: High iron content, affects liver function and the health of related organs. Great blood builder. Contains Vitamins A and C, manganese and nickel.

BLESSED THISTLE: Used to cure leg ulcers, breast cancer. Good for all organs of body, especially heart and brain, excellent for all female conditions. General tonic contains: B complex vitamins, manganese, calcium, iron, phosphorous and potassium.

RED RASPBERRY: Raspberry leaf tempers the effects of hormonal runaway, such as might occur during menstruation, pregnancy and delivery. It also relaxes uterine muscles.

SQUAW VINE: Strengthens the uterus.

MARSHMALLOW ROOT: High in calcium.

High points of this type of formulation would be additional:

PANTOTHENIC ACID: To fortify the body in dealing with stress.
CHOLINE / INOSITOL: For cholesterol reduction.
NIACINAMIDE: For opening arteries and allowing more blood to flow to vital organs and extremities (toes, fingers, eyes, and scalp).

Knowing that you can find these nutrients in a formula that will deliver most of the prime ingredients, here is how I recommend to take them: 3 at breakfast or 2 in the morning, 1 at lunch.

Acne and Skin Problems

Great for ACNE, ECZEMA, PSORIASIS and any other type of skin disturbance.

Acne has different causes. One major factor is the diet and another is surface bacteria.

In reality, it is the diet that creates the initial problem and an environment for the bacteria to flourish. With that in mind, the first step is to "clean-up" the diet by removing fatty and fried foods. Also, foods with hydrogenated fats/oils should be eliminated.

An increase to more healthful foods such as fresh fruits and vegetables, natural juices and herbal teas.

The second step is to clean-up the blood system by removing the toxins. This is accomplished with herbs.

Another step is to bring into the system, nutrients that will "feed" the skin at cellular levels so that new healthy tissue can be built.

The following program PROVIDES NUTRIENTS FOR CELLULAR REBUILDING OF THE SKIN in all conditions that require such rebuilding to enhance the appearance of the skin. INCREASES AMOUNT OF FLOW AND BLOOD through capillaries. Assists body in REMOVAL OF TOXINS FROM THE BLOOD.

Here is a formula that is available in the marketplace today that would be beneficial for providing most of the nutritional support for this condition:

Vitamin A (fish liver Oil)
Vitamin E (D-Alpha Tocopherol)
Vitamin F
Zinc (Amino Acid Chelate)
Niacin
Red Clover
Burdock Root
Dandelion Root

Here is how the nutrients work in the body:

VITAMINS

VITAMINS A & E: Feed the skin at cellular levels.
VITAMIN F: Helps to dissolve fatty deposits in the blood.
NIACIN: Opens up capillaries and provides fresh, clean and wholesome blood to face, neck and back.

HERBS

RED CLOVER, BURDOCK ROOT: Herbal blood purifiers.
DANDELION ROOT: Stimulates liver, improves digestion, cleanses.

Knowing that you can find these nutrients in a formula that will deliver most of the prime ingredients, here is how I recommend to take them:

For severe condition — 1 tablet every 3 or 4 hours for the first three (3) days then 1 tablet every meal.

SPECIAL DIETARY CONSIDERATIONS

ELIMINATE all fried, fatty and greasy foods and caffeine containing products.

INCREASE celery, garlic, carrots, spinach, all fresh and raw vegetables and fruits, sprouted seeds, whole grain products, millet, brown rice.

DRINK plenty of distilled or spring water, fresh squeezed lemon juice and water, comfrey tea, burdock tea.

EXERCISE by standing on head or use inversion devices to bring more blood to the head.

Allergies

Webster's Dictionary states that an allergy is: "exaggerated or abnormal reaction to substances, situations, or physical states, harmless to most people."

Based on that statement, it might be said that people who suffer from allergies are nutritionally or biochemically different than most people. Apparently, some bio-chemical transactions within the body may not be working effectively. This may indicate a need for additional nutritional support.

Some people who have allergic reactions have benefited from nutrients in extra amounts beyond the normal "1-A-Day".

The following program has been constructed with this understanding in mind, and it provides NATURAL ANTIHISTAMINES. Strengthens and stimulates adrenal, liver and pancreas functions. NOTE: People with allergies will generally have hypoglycemia and possibly candida albicans.

Here is a formula that is available in the marketplace today that would be beneficial for providing most of the nutritional support for this condition:

Vitamin C
Pantothenic Acid
Vitamin E (D-Alpha Tocopherol)
Manganese (amino acid chelate)
Bee Pollen
Garlic
Goldenseal Root
Ginger Root
Juniper Berries
Dandelion Root

Here is how the nutrients work in the body:

VITAMINS

VITAMIN C: Acts as natural antihistamine and detoxifier.
VITAMIN E: Has antihistamine properties.
PANTOTHENIC ACID: Strengthens adrenal glands to secrete necessary hormones.

HERBS

BEE POLLEN: Strengthens resistance to airborne contaminants.
GARLIC: Strengthens lungs and resistance to airborne contaminants.
GOLDENSEAL ROOT, GINGER, JUNIPER BERRIES: Nourish and stimulate pancreas.
DANDELION ROOT: Stimulates liver. The liver and pancreas both secrete digestive enzymes.

Knowing that you can find these nutrients in a formula that that will deliver most of the prime ingredients, here is how I recommend to take them:

For severe attack: 1 tablet every hour for first two days, then 1 tablet every two to three hours for the next two days, then 1 tablet every meal.

For general use: 1 tablet every meal.

SPECIAL DIETARY CONSIDERATIONS

ELIMINATE all allergy producing foods, and dairy products when congested.

INCREASE the intake of bee pollen / flower pollen, garlic.

DRINK plenty of licorice tea, and or dandelion root tea, distilled water, 1 / 2 fresh squeezed lemon with warm water in mornings.

Alzheimer's Disease

See MEMORY PROBLEMS : PROGRAM M-RE.

Arthritis

& Other Inflammatory Diseases

Such as ARTHRITIS (all types) and LUPUS.

Arthritis is just one of many different types of inflammatory conditions that is classified as a degenerative disease.

There are two main types of arthritis, RHEUMATOID and OSTEOARTHRITIS.

Most of the diseases that are classified as degenerative disease have no known cause according to the Merck Manual.The Merck Manual is the doctor's "bible" and lists every known ailment that affects mankind. It also includes the causes, symptoms and the recommended drugs for dealing with the problem.

In working with arthritis from a natural healing point of view we are going to take a medical approach. By that we mean we are going to deal with the symptoms first, and then look at the probable causes. The first sign that we will deal with is the inflammation.

The inflammation in this particular case is found in the joints of the body, such as, the knuckles, wrists, finger and toe joints, ankles and knees. Arthritis has also been known to effect the spine, neck and hips as well.

Since the inflammation of these various joints cause pain, an immediate goal in treating this condition would be to reduce the inflammation as quickly as possible. This would lessen the pain that is caused by the swollen tissues or joints rubbing together and would begin to bring relief from the pain almost immediately.

There are different ways to reduce the inflammation. Since we are taking a natural approach to healing this condition we need to understand the nutritional make up of arthritis, which reflects a state of imbalance in the body.

It is interesting to note that arthritics are deficient in potassium which is used by the body to regulate the balance of fluids within the cells. When there is a diminished amount of potassium there is generally an increase in sodium. Sodium forces the body to retain fluids. This retention is what causes the cells to become swollen with fluids, thus creating an inflamed condition.

Another aspect of arthritis is calcium deposits that form at the joint sites. These are often referred to as "spurs". The calcium deposits or "spurs" may develop because the uric acid levels are very high and calcium is a mineral that requires acidity for absorption. Yet within the digestive process there is not enough hydrochloric acid or amino acids, from proteins, present that are necessary for the calcium to be properly utilized, so ions of calcium float in the blood stream and are deposited in the joints as well as the arterial walls. So another goal would be to try and dissolve these calcium spurs and have the body reassimilate the calcium into the muscles where it is needed.

Research has also demonstrated that arthritics are deficient in histidine, an amino acid. Many other nutrients such as vitamin B6, pantothenic acid, magnesium, to name a few are also needed in extra amounts.

In some medical circles, arthritis is being examined as a viral disease that has been able to flourish because of the body's lowered defenses. This is brought on by a lowered immune system. As research looks at this aspect of the disease it is becoming very clear that stress is a major factor in the lowering of the body's immune system.

Stress taxes the adrenal glands which secrete hormones that carry messages to the other glands on how and/or what to perform or manufacture. All of the glands of the body are tied together in a complicated system. Each and every aspect of life within the body is dependent on each other. This is why it is so important to maintain a proper nutritional balance within. In this way you are providing the system with the needed ingredients to function correctly and thus provide optimum health. It also eliminates the opportunity for disease to take hold.

With all these factors in mind an ideal synergistically complete combination of nutrients and herbs has been created to deal effectively with the known deficiencies that arthritics suffer from.

Here is what that program will do for you: It will assist the body in REDUCING INFLAMMATION IN THE JOINTS; DISSOLVING CALCIUM DEPOSITS; NEUTRALIZING THE ACIDITY OF THE BLOOD; IT IMPROVES CIRCULATION; INCREASES THE BODY'S THRESHOLD FOR PAIN; IMPROVES THE BODY'S RESISTANCE TO STRESS AND INFECTION.

Here is a formula that is available in the marketplace today that would be beneficial for providing most of the nutritional support for this condition:

Vitamin B6
Pantothenic Acid (B5)
Niacinamide
Vitamin D (Fish Liver Oil)
DL-Phenylalanine
L-Histidine(Free Form Amino Acid)
Raw Adrenal
Raw Thymus
Potassium(Amino Acid Complex)
Magnesium(Amino Acid Chelate)
Bromelin(Natural Pineapple)
Yucca
Alfalfa
Chaparral
Hydrangea   Celery Seed
Uva Ursi   Fennel Seed
Corn Silk   White Willow Bark

Here is how the nutrients work in the body:

VITAMINS
VITAMIN B6: To reduce water content and inflammation.
PANTOTHENIC ACID: Feeds the adrenal glands which are the stress centers.
VITAMIN D: Assists the body in assimilating calcium.
NIACINAMIDE: Opens arteries and improves blood flow.

MINERALS
POTASSIUM: To regulate water balance and acid alkaline balance in the blood.
MAGNESIUM: For calcium assimilation.

HERBS
ALFALFA AND CELERY SEEDS: Reduce acidity and inflammation.
YUCCA AND CHAPARRAL: The saponin in them acts as a lubricant in the joints.
HYDRANGEA, CORNSILK, UVA URSI: Excellent diuretic herbs for reducing inflammation.

OTHER SYNERGISTIC NUTRIENTS
HISTIDINE: An amino acid that is usually lacking in people who suffer from arthritis.
RAW THYMUS: To stimulate the immune system.
RAW ADRENAL: To stimulate adrenal activity.
DL-PHENYLALANINE: Nutrient that deals with pain.

Knowing that you can find these nutrients in a formula that will deliver most of the prime ingredients, here is how I recommend to take them:

For severe conditions (stiffness, pain, inflammation): 1 tablet every hour for the first day, then 1 tablet every two hours for the next two days, then 1 tablet every three hours for two days, then 1 every meal.

SPECIAL DIETARY CONSIDERATIONS
ELIMINATE tomatoes, eggplant, oranges, grapefruit, all white flour products, fried foods, meat, chicken (reduced if not omitted), preservatives and artificial colors/ flavors, sugar, salt.
INCREASE the consumption of raw vegetables — carrots, celery, parsley, cucumbers, garlic, potatoes, alfalfa sprouts. Fresh fruits — bananas, peaches, pears, watermelon, plums, red grapes, cherries, papaya, pineapple. Whole grains — buckwheat, millet, soybeans.
DRINK plenty of corn silk tea. Alfalfa tea would be good.

Asthma

See CONGESTION AND SINUS PROBLEMS : PROGRAM M-DEG

Backaches

See OSTEOPOROSIS : PROGRAM M / OS.

Blood Cleansing
PROGRAM-HE / F

Good in all situations that detoxification is necessary. Excellent when used in combination with Formulas M-DER; M-DER / l; M-PSO / s; M-VR / s to clear up such conditions as: acne, eczema, psoriasis, warts, fungal infections.

The importance of a solid internal cleansing program can not be stressed enough. To begin with everything you eat, drink or breathe ends up in your blood stream. Not all of it but enough to cause problems if left to accumulate over the years.

Once in the blood stream the pollutants, more commonly referred to as toxins, pass through the liver, lungs, kidneys and intestinal tract. In each organ that blood passes through it deposits some of these toxins, as well as, picks up the newest ones that enter into the system. Each organ or system mentioned also acts as a filtering plant to remove the toxins from the blood stream. However this is not always effective because there is often more coming in than is being removed. So we must take specific steps to purify our internal systems and make them truly FIT to deal with the future toxins.

When trying to create a fit cleansing system it becomes necessary to work on many areas. To gain the most benefit in the shortest period of time it would be wise to work on the liver and the blood at the same time.

Here is a formula that is available in the marketplace today that would be beneficial for providing most of the nutritional support for this condition:

Burdock Root
Red Clover
Gotu Kola
Echinacea
Yellow Dock
Stillingia Root
Chaparral

Here is how the herbs work in the body:

BURDOCK ROOT: All around blood purifier, strongly diuretic and diaphoretic. Cleanse the body of toxins, markedly enhances liver and gall/bile functions.

RED CLOVER: In Europe, used extensively as a diuretic to treat gout.

GOTU KOLA: Blood purifier, glandular tonic, diuretic.

ECHINACEA: Significantly stimulates the body's own blood cleaning system. Destroys the germs of infection directly, bolsters the body's defenses by magnifying the white blood cell count, Echinacin, the active constituent of Echinacea, interferon-like activity. It protects cells against virus related diseases, such as herpes, influenza, canker sores, etc.

YELLOW DOCK: Primarily affects liver function and the health of related organs, increasing their ability to strain and purify the blood. In addition, the herb has antibacterial properties. High iron content, high thiamine content.

Knowing that you can find these nutrients in a formula that will deliver most of the prime ingredients, here is how I recommend to take them: 1 or 2 at each meal. This depends on need, progress and results.

SPECIAL DIETARY CONSIDERATIONS

ELIMINATE as much of the preseravtives, food colorings and additives as possible. Tap water. Meats that are not well prepared or cooked.

INCREASE celery, onions, garlic, carrots, parsley and as much raw vegtables and fresh fruit as possible.

DRINK clean distilled water throughout the day. Chaparral tea or any of the herbs in this formula that can be found as a tea.

Candida Albicans

Today's health picture is overshadowed by a condition called Candida Albicans, a technical term for a yeast infection. Actually, I don't believe it to be an "infection" as much as it is a "colonization of the host environment".

The yeast bacteria are able to flourish within the body because it provides a friendly atmosphere for growth. This atmosphere is the result of a weakened immune system and lack of "friendly" bacteria in the intestinal tract. This "lack" has been brought about by the indiscriminate use of medicinal drugs.

In order for the body to free itself of this infestation, it must become nutritionally fit. This means a strong immune system and a "hostile" environment for the yeast bacteria.

Creating a hostile environment means depriving the yeast colony of its food sources and attacking them full force with natural substances that will destroy them and at the same time strengthen and stimulate the immune system to "clean house".

This nutritional program is designed to DESTROY BACTERIA, STIMULATES IMMUNE SYSTEM and INCREASES ELIMINATION OF TOXINS.

When you work with this program it is important to follow the dietary guidelines. In this way you cut off the food supply to the "yeast" and speed recovery.

Here is a formula that is available in the marketplace today that would be beneficial for providing most of the nutritional support for this condition:

Garlic	Buckthorn Bark
Pau D'Arco	Zinc(Amino Acid Chelate)
Black Walnut	Vitamin A(Fish Liver Oil)
Dandelion Root	Pantothenic Acid
Myrrh	Vitamin B1(Thiamine)
Echinacea	Vitamin B2(Riboflavin)
Goldenseal Root	Vitamin B6(Pyridoxine)
Corn Silk	Biotin
Uva Ursi	L-Cysteine(Amino Acid)
Cascara Sagrada	Acidophilus(Carrot source)

Here is how the nutrients work in the body:

VITAMINS

VITAMIN A: Nourishes the thymus gland. Increases its size and antibody production.

VITAMIN B1, B2, B6: Involved in nourishing the adrenal glands. It is necessary to do this because when the body is sick or under attack it creates stress. Stress runs down the adrenal glands. When the adrenal glands are taxed and depleted they stress out and deplete the immune system. Thus without feeding them you prolong any illness that the body is dealing with.

PANTOTHENIC ACID: Nourishes the adrenal glands.

HERBS

GOLDENSEAL ROOT, MYRRH, PAU D'ARCO, BLACK WALNUT: Known to contain natural properties that kill bacteria.

ECHINACEA: Cleanses lymph system and improves antibody production.

DANDELION: Improves function of liver. Bile and certain enzymes produced in the liver aid in maintaining proper intestinal flora.

CORN SILK, UVA URSI, CASCARA SAGRADA AND BUCKTHORN BARK: Help in cleansing the system of toxic and waste material.

OTHER SYNERGISTIC NUTRIENTS

L-CYSTEINE: Involved in anti-body production.

ZINC: Essential for anti-body production.

Knowing that you can find these nutrients in a formula that will deliver most of the prime ingredients, here is how I recommend to take them:

For severe condition: 1 tablet every 2 hours for the first day. 2 tablets each meal and before bed the second day. 1 tablet each meal and before bed until bottle is empty.

SPECIAL DIETARY CONSIDERATIONS
YEAST CONTROL DIET

Foods You Can Eat

All Fresh Vegetables

Asparagus	Green Peppers	Squash	Mustard
Beets	Onions	White Potatoes	Beet
Broccoli	Parsley	Sweet Potatoes	Collard
Brussels Sprouts	Peas, Beans and	Radishes	Kale
Cabbage	Legumes	Okra	Lettuce
Carrots	Tomatoes, Fresh	Parsnip	
Cauliflower	Summer and	Corn	
Celery	Winter Squash,	Greens	
Cucumbers	Zucchini, Acorn	Turnip	
Eggplant	and Butternut	Spinach	

All Fresh Fruits

Apples	Peach	Berries (all)	Orange
Avocado	Pear	Cherries	Papaya
Banana	Pineapple	Mango	Plum
Grapes	Apricot	Nectarine	

Meat and Eggs

(any but bacon, sausage, ham, hot dogs or luncheon meats.)

Beef (limit)	Egg	Lobster	Rabbit
Chicken	Tuna	Shrimp	Quail
Turkey	Salmon and other	Crab	Duck
Lamb	fresh Fish	Oysters	Goose
Veal	Clams	Squirrel	Cornish Hen

Pheasant and other game birds

Nuts, Seeds & Oils
Unprocessed

Almonds	Filberts
Brazil Nuts	Pecans
Cashews	Pumpkin Seeds

Oils (cold pressed)

Almond	Olive
Apricot	Safflower
Avocado	Sesame
Corn	Sunflower
Linseed	Butter

Whole Grains

Barley	Oats
Corn	Rice
Millet	Wheat

Cereal Grains, and Muffins (containing no yeast, honey or sugar)

Beverages

Milk
Water

YEAST CONTROL DIET

Foods You Cannot Eat

A. Sugar and sugar containing foods: sucrose, fructose, mulattoes, lactose glycogen, glucose, mannitol, sorbitol, galactose, mono-saccharide and polysaccharide. Also avoid honey, molasses, maple syrup, date sugar and turbinado sugar.

B. Yeast, breads and pastries.

C. Alcoholic beverages: wine, beer, whiskey, brandy, gin, rum, vodka, etc. Also fermented beverages such as cider and rootbeer.

D. Malt products.

E. Condiments, sauces and vinegar containing foods: mustard, ketchup, Worcestershire, Accent, etc. Also horseradish, mince meat, tamari and sauerkraut.

F. Processed and smoked meats.

G. Dried and candied fruits.

H. Leftovers: mold often grows on leftover foods that are refrigerated. Freezing is best.

I. Fruit juices.

J. Coffee and tea: includes herb teas.

K. Melons.

L. Edible Fungi: all types of mushrooms.

M. Cheeses: also buttermilk, sour cream and sour milk.

N. Yeast: Brewer's yeast and baker's yeast.

O. Vitamins and mineral that contain yeast.

P. Nuts: Peanuts and pistachios usually contain mold.

Cataracts

Three-fifths of all people between the ages of 65 and 74 show the beginning signs of cataracts, and by age 80 nearly everyone's vision is clouded by them to some degree.

Surgery to remove and replace lenses of the eye damaged by cataracts is the most frequently performed operation in the U.S. — 650,000 of them annually, costing a whopping one billion dollars! If preventive measures could be taken to delay cataract formations by the average of 10 years, notes *Discover* magazine (Feb. 1984), then the number of operations could be cut in half.

Various types of stress usually cause cataracts. Besides the aging process itself, illnesses like diabetes also account for a lost of cataracts. Frequent exposure to x-rays or microwaves, to intense heat from blast furnaces or welding torches, or even to the ultraviolet rays of the sun are also known causes.

Protein and vitamin deficiencies can be a contributing factor. So can drugs like cortisone, or a severe blow to the eye. More common causes, though, suggests the *Journal of The American Dietetic Association* (March 1985) are insufficient levels of fluids such as water in the body and the excessive consumption of milk in later adulthood.

Minerals and vitamins can prevent diabetic cataracts, reported *The New England Journal of Medicine* (Jan. 5th, 1978). Chief among those recommended are calcium and magnesium and all vitamins from the B-complex group. Additionally, vitamin A is very important to keep the eyes from drying out, says *Science News* (Oct. 13th, 1984). Finally, vitamin C and especially its bioflavonoids can prevent cataracts, reports the journal *Science* (Jan. 14th, 1977). The sulphur amino acid, glutathione, likewise protects against cataracts, claim Drs. Braverman and Pfeiffer in their *Healing Nutrients Within* (Keats, 1987).

Here is a formula that is available in the marketplace today that would be beneficial for providing most of the nutritional support for this condition:

VITAMIN A (fish liver oil)	SELENIUM
VITAMIN D (fish liver oil)	ZINC
VITAMIN E (d alpha tocopherol)	PAPAYOTIN
VITAMIN B1(Thiamine)	BROMELIN
VITAMIN B2 (Riboflavine)	PANCREATIN
VITAMIN B6(Pyridoxine)	L-GLYCINE
VITAMIN B12(Cobalamin)	L-GLUTAMINE
INOSITOL	L-ARGININE
FOLIC ACID (Folacin)	L-CYSTEINE HCL
NIACIN(Nicotinic Acid)	L-GLUTATHIONE
PANTOTHENIC ACID	EYEBRIGHT
VITAMIN C (Ascorbic Acid)	CHICKWEED
BIOFLAVONOID (Vitamin P)	CARDAMON
CALCIUM (Amino Acid Chelate)	GINGER
MAGNESIUM	RED RASPBERRY LEAVES

Here are the nutrients and why they help:

VITAMINS

VITAMIN A: Formation of rich blood, maintenance of good eyesight. Essential in the formation of visual purple, a substance in the eye which is necessary for proper night vision.

VITAMIN E: Vitamin E is an antioxidant. As a diuretic, vitamin E helps lower elevated blood pressure. Protects against the damaging effects of many environmental poisons in the air, water and food.

VITAMIN B1 (Thiamine): Thiamine, essential for proper nerve function.

VITAMIN B2 (Riboflavin): Cataracts can easily be produced in laboratory animals by depriving them of riboflavin. So diets deficient in vitamin C can produce scurvy. These same diets can also produce cataracts. A diet low in protein has also been linked to this eye disorder. A deficiency of riboflavin can cause anemia, visual fatigue, a "sandy" feeling of the eyes, inability to endure bright lights. Seborrhea, a scaly skin disease, is also a symptom of riboflavin deficiency.

VITAMIN B6 (Pyridoxine): Getting enough of the B vitamin would help to prevent raised cholesterol levels. Those patients with hardening of the arteries were found to have very low levels of pyridoxine in their blood.

VITAMIN B12: Helps iron function better, aids folic acid in the synthesis of choline. Helps the placement of vitamin A into body tissues by aiding carotene absorption or vitamin A conversion. It has been used with some success in treating Glaucoma, treating this condition by injecting vitamin B12. A Japanese physician has confirmed the Russian findings by giving one milligram of vitamin B12.

INOSITOL: Inositol is closely related in function to the B vitamins choline and biotin.

VITAMIN B3 (Niacin): Niacin appears to reduce the level of cholesterol in the blood. The large doses of niacin brought about a reduction in cholesterol without any change in diet. It also provides more blood to all areas of the body.

VITAMIN C (Ascorbic Acid): protects thiamine, riboflavin, folic acid, pantothenic acid, and vitamin A and E against oxidation.

BIOFLAVONOID (Vitamin P): The components of the bioflavonoid are citrin, hesperidin, rutin, flavones, and flavonals. Essential for the proper absorption and use of vitamin C.

PANTOTHENIC ACID (B5): Essential constituent of coenzyme A, which forms active acetate and, as such, acts as an activating agent in metabolism.

MINERALS

CALCIUM: Calcium assists in the process of blood clotting and helps prevent the accumulation of too much acid or too much alkali in the blood.

MAGNESIUM: Magnesium activates more enzymes in the body than any other mineral.

ZINC: The vascular coating of the eye contains more zinc than any other part of the body. Zinc is essential for the treatment of arteriosclerosis. Zinc is essential, it seems, to "mobilize" vitamin A from the liver, so that it can perform its usual bodily functions.

SELENIUM: Is a natural antioxidant and appears to preserve elasticity of tissue by delaying oxidation of polyunsaturated fatty acids.

AMINO ACIDS

L-GLUTAMINE: Can readily cross the blood-barrier into the brain where it is quickly converted into glutamic acid. Serves primarily as a fuel for the brain which also keeps excess amounts of ammonia from damaging the brain.

L-CYSTEINE HCL: Involved in antibody production.

L-GLUTATHIONE: Protects the lens metabolism by preserving the physicochemical equilibrium of lens proteins, maintains the molecular integrity of the lens fiber membranes, protects membranes and organelles from oxidation.

HERBS

EYEBRIGHT: Sore and / or inflamed eyes.

CHICKWEED: Hemorrhoids, eye infections, (glaucoma, cataracts), blood diseases (leukemia, tetanus), and eczema.

RED RASPBERRY LEAVES: Astringent on the eyes (reducing mucous in them), hyperglycemia (abnormal amounts of glucose in the blood), cataracts that may be related to it.

Knowing that you can find these nutrients in a formula that will deliver most of the prime ingredients, here is how I recommend to take them: 2 or 3 tablets at each meal depending on the degree of vision difficulty.

SPECIAL DIETARY CONSIDERATIONS

ELIMINATE all fried foods, fatty meats and most dairy products, white flour, sugar and salt.

INCREASE the consumption of raw vegetables especially carrots, yams, spinach, celery, endives and fresh fruits, anise, papaya, pineapple, apples, grapefruit, lemon juice, garlic, onions, dark leafy greens.

DRINK 2 tablespoons flax seed oil daily, dandelion tea, gotu kola tea, and specifically eyebright tea. Carrot juice mixed with endives and a dash of parsley would also be very beneficial.

Poor Circulation _____

Excellent as a ORAL CHELATION program. Beneficial for people suffering from hair loss, hearing problems, numb and tingling extremities, arms and legs that frequently fall asleep, poor memory. This program should be used in all situations requiring improved blood flow.

The circulatory system is the lifeline of the body. It carries the oxygen and food (vitamins, minerals, fats, proteins, and fuel (blood sugars) that our body requires for health and performance. A "well fed" body is a healthy and vibrant body.

The way to insure that all the organs, muscles, nerves and skin remain well fed is to keep the lifelines (arteries) open and free flowing. Problems begin when the arteries begin to clog and diminish the amount of blood available to all necessary points.

The process of clogging takes place when excess fats/cholesterol abound in the blood stream. They begin to clump together forming larger and larger fatty deposits. As they grow in size, they capture minute particles of minerals (ions) that are floating in the blood stream. This begins a "hardening" process, a situation where the fatty deposits begin to cling to the arterial walls. This can lead to arteriosclerosis hardening of the arteries.

So if we are to avoid circulatory problems, we must first identify the symptoms. This will help to determine if we do have a potential circulatory and eventual heart problem.

The symptoms of poor circulation are generally:

1. Hair loss
2. Memory loss
3. Hearing loss
4. Cold hands and feet
5. Numbness in fingers and toes
6. Arms and legs that "fall asleep" easily.

If we have three (3) or more of these symptoms it's time to take action. To open up our arteries and let the blood flow.

One step of our actions should be to reduce the intake of those foods that contribute to excess fat/cholesterol in our blood. Remember the fat/cholesterol is the "cement" that binds the minerals in our blood to the arterial walls.

The second step would be to start a nutritional program that will dissolve the fat/cholesterol deposits that currently exist. This would then improve the flow of blood to our heart, head, hands and feet.

With these considerations in mind the following program was created to perform the following functions: OPEN ARTERIES, DISSOLVE CHOLESTEROL and TRI-GLYCERIDE, REDUCE WATER CONTENT,

REASSIMILATE CALCIUM FROM ARTERIAL WALLS, REGULATE CHOLESTEROL, EQUALIZE BLOOD PRESSURE AND TONE THE HEART.

Here is a formula that is available in the marketplace today that would be beneficial for providing most of the nutritional support for this condition:

Choline
Inositol
L-Methionine (Free Form Amino Acid)
Vitamin B6 (Pyridoxine)
Vitamin F (Unsaturated Fatty Acids)
Vitamin D (Fish Liver Oil)
Niacinamide
Pantothenic Acid (B5)
Betaine HCL
Magnesium (Amino Acid Chelate)
Apple Pectin
Hawthorne Berry
Garlic
Capsicum
Ginger

Here is how the nutrients work in the body:

VITAMINS

NIACINAMIDE: Excellent for opening up arteries and in doing so provides more blood and oxygen to heart, head and extremities.

CHOLINE, INOSITOL: These are lipotropic nutrients which work as "fat burners" dissolving excess fat and cholesterol.

VITAMIN F: Unsaturated fatty acids are essential for the dissolving of cholesterol and saturated fats in the blood stream.

VITAMIN B6: As a natural diuretic, reduces water and water pressure from the cardiovascular system. Excellent in metabolizing fats, proteins and carbohydrates.

VITAMIN D: Also essential for calcium assimilation. Most people with poor circulation are also calcium starved. This is the result of the calcium being lodged in the cholesterol plaque in the arteries.

HERBS

APPLE PECTIN: Helps to regulate cholesterol and also draws toxic metals out of the blood. It is said that apple pectin contains electro-magnetic properties.

HAWTHORNE BERRY: Added because of its heart strengthening properties.

GARLIC, CAPSICUM AND GINGER: Stimulate and purify the blood. Increase flow and regulate blood pressure.

OTHER SYNERGISTIC NUTRIENTS

METHIONINE: Is an amino acid that acts as a "fat burner". It is essential in the production of lecithin.

MAGNESIUM and HYDROCHLORIC ACID: For calcium assimilation.

Knowing that you can find these nutrients in a formula that will deliver most of the prime ingredients, here is how I recommend to take them:

For severe condition: (blue fingers/toes), constant numbness in fingers/toes: 1 tablet every hour and 2 before bed for the first 3 days then, 2 tablets each meal thereafter.

For regular conditions: 2 tablets each meal.

SPECIAL DIETARY CONSIDERATIONS

ELIMINATE all fried foods, fatty meats and most dairy products, white flour, sugar and salt.

INCREASE the consumption of raw vegetables and fresh fruits, anise, papaya, pineapple, apples, grapefruit, lemon juice, garlic, onions, artichokes, watercress, okra, dark leafy greens.

DRINK 2 tablespoons flax seed oil daily, dandelion tea, gotu kola tea, and/or ginseng tea.

Colds, Flues and Infections

Excellent for all INFECTIONS that are active within the body.

Many of us seem to separate colds and flues from infections thinking that infections are much stronger in their attack on the body. The truth of the matter is that colds and flues ARE infections. The three of them all start from the same source, a germ, virus or other form of bacteria.

The major difference is that colds and flues are generally short lived. We approach dealing with them from a different point of view than we do when we are treating an infection.

However the best way to deal with all of them, regardless of the type of infection, is the same way. Attack them head on by strengthening the immune system and fortifying the antibodies with the nutritional help that they require to function correctly. In addition to that, bring into the system those herbs that are known to kill germs on contact. Herbs such as GARLIC and GOLDENSEAL ROOT.

Using these two herbs in combination with the proper nutrients WILL speed your body to recovery regardless of what the infection. Obviously the CORRECT amount of each nutrient is necessary.

The body is the true healer. Through it's own DIVINE INTELLIGENCE the body knows what to do. All that nutrition does is provide the body with the correct materials that are needed to perform the functions that will destroy invaders. This is easily verified by the type of doctor who is willing to let you know that the drugs are not the healing agents but are only given to lessen the attack. In some instances they are only effective for reducing the symptoms while your body does the healing.

So then, what exactly is needed by the body to eliminate a cold, flu or infection? The answer begins with the immune system, specifically the thymus gland. The thymus is considered the power seat of the immune system. But in addition to nourishing the thymus we must also work on the adrenal at the very same time because the adrenal glands affect the immune system.

When the body is getting sick, or is already sick it is under stress, and stress taxes the immune system.

With all these factors in mind an ideal synergistically complete nutritional program has been created to assist your body in dealing with the invading germs.

Here is how that program works in the body: IT STRENGTHENS THE IMMUNE SYSTEM and ADRENAL GLANDS. INCREASES ANTIBODY PRODUCTION, AND KILLS BACTERIA ON CONTACT.

When any type of infection is present, it is always best to eat as much fresh and raw foods as possible. A rule of thumb is:

FRUITS CLEANSE; VEGETABLES HEAL

Here is a formula that is available in the marketplace today that would be beneficial for providing most of the nutritional support for this condition:

Vitamin A (fish liver oil)   Goldenseal Root
Vitamin C (with rose hips)   Pantothenic Acid
Garlic (powder concentrate)   Zinc (amino acid chelate)

Here is how the nutrients work in the body:

VITAMINS

VITAMIN A: Nourishes, stimulates and increases the size and effectiveness of the Thymus gland, the power center of the immune system.

VITAMIN C: A natural cold fighter because it helps to increase the number of white blood cells.

PANTOTHENIC ACID: Nourishes the adrenal glands, which are taxed because of the stress of infection in the body.

HERBS

GARLIC: Most used herb as a natural antibiotic.

GOLDENSEAL ROOT: Another herb with germicidal action and is employed by knowledgeable herbalists everywhere.

OTHER SYNERGISTIC NUTRIENTS

ZINC: Strengthens the immune system. Knowing that you can find these nutrients in a formula that will deliver most of the prime ingredients, here is how I recommend to take them:

For infections (adults): 1 or 2 every hour for 2 days, then 1 or 2 every two hours for 2 days, infection or cold should be terminated or greatly reduced. **NOTE:** Adults can take up to 30 tablets daily for 3 to 4 days.

For infections (children): 1 every 2-3 hours for 4 days, then 1 every 3-4 hours, if needed. **NOTE:** Children can take up to 10-15 tablets daily for 3 to 4 days.

SPECIAL DIETARY CONSIDERATIONS

ELIMINATE all solid foods if fever is present.

INCREASE intake of vitamin C, A, B6, garlic, bioflavonoids, honey, rose hips, fresh juices and some raw seeds, nuts and sprouted seeds and grains. Include hot epsom salt baths, plenty of rest, mild excercises, and walking in fresh air.

DRINK when fever is present only drink fresh fruit and vegetables juices, diluted with water plus herb teas. Other juices are lemon, black currant, orange, pineapple, elderberries (particularly for bronchial catarrh), carrot, beet, tomato, green pepper, watercress, plus onion and garlic juice in small amounts added to vegetable juices.

Lung Congestion

Pure herbal decongestant that is ideal for ALL LUNG CONGESTION (regardless of cause), including EMPHYSEMA and ASTHMA.

Generally speaking, temporary lung congestion is usually the result of a cold or flu. For some people it is brought on by smoking (emphysema) or emotional stress (asthma) or allergies. In each and every instance the condition is the same, lungs full of phlegm and mucus.

The goal in such a condition is to break up the congestion, the phlegm and mucus and get it out of the lungs. Fortunately there are specific herbs that can perform that feat with little effort.

The herbs BREAK UP MUCUS AND PHLEGM CONGESTION AND FACILITATE QUICK REMOVAL. Excellent for colds, allergies, asthma, emphysema.

Here is a formula that is available in the marketplace today that would be beneficial for providing most of the nutritional support for this condition:

Comfrey Root   Mullein
Fenugreek   Thyme
Slippery Elm

Here is how these herbs work in the body:

COMFREY AND MULLEIN: Break up mucus and phlegm.
FENUGREEK AND THYME: Have germicidal properties.
SLIPPERY ELM: Excellent for pulling mucus out.

Knowing that you can find these nutrients in a formula that will deliver most of the prime ingredients, here is how I recommend to take them:

For heavy congestion, asthma attacks, emphysema: 1 tablet every hour for the first two days, then 1 tablet every two hours for the next two (2) to three (3) days, then 1 or 2 every meal and 1 before bed. For light to moderate congestion: 1 tablet every 2 hours for the first 2 days, then 1 or 2 every meal and before bed. For basic maintenance: 1 tablet in the morning and/or 1 in the evening depending on patients history of congestion.

SPECIAL DIETARY CONSIDERATIONS

ELIMINATE all dairy products, white flour products, sugar and starches.

INCREASE vegetables — parsley, carrots, celery, beets, garlic, onions, cucumbers, green leafy vegetables. Fruits — apples, apricots, bananas, pineapple, blueberries, Also include buckwheat, peas, beans. Nuts — almond, brazil. Bee pollen as granules or tablets.

DRINK rose hip tea, horehound tea. One (1) teaspoon fresh squeezed lime juice as needed to cut mucus.

Constipation

See LAXATIVE : PROGRAM M-LA.

Cramps

See OSTEOPOROSIS : PROGRAM M/OS.

Diabetes
PROGRAM M-DIB

Excellent for DIABETES. Able to reduce and possibly eliminate insulin dependence. Careful management is essential. Diabetes is the name of a condition that deals with poor "sugar" metabolism. The sugar in question is really called glucose. It is a by-product of carbohydrates and it is used by the body as a fuel.

To help us metabolize (burn) glucose, the pancreas produces insulin. When the amount of insulin produced is inadequate to burn the sugar in the blood, you then have the condition called diabetes (excessive glucose in the blood). Diabetes is characterized by: Excessive Thirst, Frequent Urination, Increased Appetite, and Loss of Weight.

There are other symptoms but these are the most common.

There are specific nutrients and herbs that can help the body metabolize blood sugar and increase its ability to produce insulin.

The following program AIDS BODY IN SUGAR METABOLISM, INCREASES INSULIN PRODUCTION, NOURISHES, STRENGTHENS AND STIMULATES PANCREAS.

Here is a formula that is available in the marketplace today that would be beneficial for providing most of the nutritional support for this condition:

GTF Chromium
Zinc (amino acid chelate)
Manganese (amino acid chelate)
Kelp
Vitamin B 1 (thiamine)
Niacinamide
Pantothenic Acid
L-Glutamine (amino acid)
Vitamin F
Raw Pancreas
Sinita Organa
Goldenseal Root

Cedar Berries
Dandelion Root
Comfrey
Blueberry Leaf
Ginger

Here is how the nutrients work in the body:

VITAMINS

VITAMIN B1: For carbohydrate metabolism.
PANTOTHENIC ACID: Nourishes adrenal glands.
NIACINAMIDE: Opens arteries — increases blood to toes / eyes.
VITAMIN F: Increases fat / glucose metabolism.

MINERALS

GTF CHROMIUM: Assists in using glucose(blood sugar).
ZINC: Helps insulin formation.
MANGANESE: Works with Chromium.
KELP: Increases metabolism.

HERBS

GOLDENSEAL ROOT: Lowers blood sugar and stimulates pancreas.
CEDAR BERRIES: Stimulates pancreas.
GINGER: Stimulates pancreas and improves blood flow.
COMFREY: Regulates blood sugar.
SINITA ORGANA: Acts as natural insulin.

OTHER SYNERGISTIC NUTRIENTS

L-GLUTAMINE: Reduces sugar craving.
RAW PANCREAS: Nourishes and stimulates pancreas.

Knowing that you can find these nutrients in a formula that will deliver most of the prime ingredients, here is how I recommend to take them: 1 tablet each meal.

SPECIAL DIETARY CONSIDERATIONS

ELIMINATE all sweets, sugar, salt, white flour products.
INCREASE nopales (cactus, this is Sinita Organa), string beans, almonds, almond butter, cucumbers, asparagus, peas, beans, buckwheat, garlic, Brewer's yeast, fresh vegetables, 2 tablespoons coldpressed vegetable oil daily, this is done to speed up the dissolving of fatty / acid material in the blood stream.
DRINK 3 cups of blueberry leaf tea on a daily basis.
EXERCISE by walking briskly, and swim.

Diarrhea

Diarrhea is a problem for both young and old. It can become dangerous in the fact that it can dehydrate the body. In addition to that there is nutrient depletion.

When the body is dealing with diarrhea, regardless of the cause, the food that has been ingested is rapidly expelled from the system. With this kind of condition taking place there is very little, if any, assimilation of nutrients from the food. So in order to avoid a major health hazard it becomes necessary to stop the diarrhea as quickly as possible.

The very best way to accomplish this task is by tackling the problem head on. Since diarrhea is more of a symptom than a disease we need to attack symptomatically.

To begin with, we need to kill whatever parasite or germ that may be the cause. Then there is the excess liquid that has to be absorbed. This will cause the bowels to become harder.

By stopping the diarrhea process, all food that is consumed will stay within the body longer affording the system the opportunity to extract whatever nutrients it needs for rebuilding the system.

In Mexico where this condition is more common, the people do two interesting things. First they squeeze fresh lemon juice over all salads before they eat them and when diarrhea does strike they eat plenty of cheese. This acts to gel the bowels.

The following herbs act as gelling and liquid absorbing agents. In doing so they are able to solidify bowels and regulate movement when diarrhea is present.

Here is a formula that is available in the marketplace today that would be beneficial for providing most of the nutritional support for this condition:

Acacia	White Oak
Carob	Bayberry
Rhubarb	Blackberry
Alum	Charcoal
Sweet Leaf	Garlic Powder
Cinnamon	Pau D'Arco

Here is how these herbs work in the body:

ACACIA AND CAROB: Absorbs discharges and soothes irritated linings of the intestines.

RHUBARB, BLACKBERRY, BAYBERRY, WHITE OAK: All are known as powerful astringent herbs used by healers in combatting diarrhea.

ALUM: Another strong gelling agent.

CHARCOAL: Absorbs liquid and excess gas.

GARLIC, PAU D'ARCO: Used to kill bacteria.

Knowing that you can find these nutrients in a formula that will deliver most of the prime ingredients, here is how I recommend to take them:

For children: If the child cannot swallow the capsules or tablets, then open the capsules or crush the tablets and mix with applesauce or banana; administer in the following way: 1 capsule every two (2) hours, watch for results so as not to cause constipation.

For adults: 1 or 2 every hour. Again watch the results.

SPECIAL DIETARY CONSIDERATIONS

ELIMINATE if it is an acute condition, all foods for three days except cooked white rice with applesauce made from raw apples. For a metabolic condition do not drink liquids with meals.

INCREASE gradually cooked vegetables, millet, whole rice and soured milks, such as buttermilk, yogurt, etc. Raw foods after condition is completely corrected. Also include bananas or papaya fruit. For a metabolic condition have small frequent meals, chew food extremely well. Cereals: brown rice, millet, oats and buckwheat.

DRINK all fresh vegetable and fruit juices. Also included is carob, dried blueberries, cinnamon 4 to 6 cups of herb tea each day. For a metabolic condition drink liquids one hour before or two hours after the meal.

Diuretic

See WATER RETENTION : PROGRAM M-WA.

Emphysema

See CONGESTION AND SINUS PROBLEMS : PROGRAM M-DEG

Energy Problems

See HYPOGLYCEMIA : PROGRAM M-PE / U.

Fertililty Problems
PROGRAMS M-FE / M; M-FE / F

Provides additional support for couples trying to become pregnant. Essential for partner diagnosed as having a weakened system.

It is astounding to realize that over 2 million young couples cannot have children because of infertility problems.

There are many causes for infertility in both the male and female. Some of the problems lie in psychological areas such as, responsibilities, not wanting to stay in the relationship, fear of parenthood. For others, it may be their career, additional stress and financial burdens. All of these psychological factors cause stress within and stress depletes the body's nutritional reserves.

Poor nutritional reserves coupled with an inadequate diet, causes even greater depletion of the essential nutrients necessary for the proper functioning of the reproductive system.

Now with these factors in mind, an ideal approach would be to replace, as efficiently as possible all of the nutrients that the body would require.

The following program provides ALL ESSENTIAL NUTRIENTS FOR THE REPRODUCTIVE SYSTEMS. NOURISHES, TONES STIMULATES and INCREASES HORMONE PRODUCTION, both male and female, SPERM COUNT and MOTILITY FACTORS in the male, STRENGTHENS OVARIES and EGG PRODUCTION.

Here is a formula that is available in the marketplace today that would be beneficial for providing most of the nutritional support for the male:

Vitamin A (Fish Liver Oil)	Selenium
Vitamin E (D-Alpha Tocopheryl)	Ginseng Root
Vitamin C (With Rose Hips)	Damiana
Vitamin B12	False Unicorn
Inositol	Saw Palmetto
Pantothenic Acid	Fenugreek
Folic Acid	Sarsaparilla
Niacinamide	Glove
Zinc (Amino Acid Chelate)	Yohimbe
Calcium (Amino Acid Chelate)	L-Glutamine (Amino Acid)
Magnesium (Amino Acid Chelate)	L-Arginine (Amino Acid)
Manganese (Amino Acid Chelate)	L-Cysteine (Amino Acid)
Sulfur (Zinc Sulphate)	L-Methionine (Amino Acid)

Here is how the nutrients work in the body:

VITAMINS

VITAMIN A: Involved in a chemical process that creates sexual hormones in both male and female.

VITAMINS C, E: Act as anti-oxidants and protect the following vitamins from destruction due to oxidation: Vitamins A, B1, Pantothenic Acid, Folic Acid and Niacin.

VITAMIN E: Works with selenium in promoting normal body growth and sexual fertility.

VITAMIN B12: Also important in the reproductive process. High amounts are found in the testes.

UNSATURATED FATTY ACIDS: Essential for normal glandular functions and activities, especially the reproductive system.

FOLIC ACID, A, C, E: Work together to produce sperm.

NIACINAMIDE: Necessary for sex hormone production and health.

PANTOTHENIC ACID: Works in maintaining sex hormone production.

MINERALS

CALCIUM, MAGNESIUM, ZINC, SULFUR: Work with B12, C and inositol as important factors in the construction of healthy sperm.

MANGANESE: Maintains sex hormone production.

ZINC: Plays a vital role in growth and development of the reproductive glands.

HERBS

GINSENG, DAMIANA, SARSAPARILLA, SAW PALMETTO AND YOHIMBE: Known for male enhancement properties, sexual rejuvenation.

AMINO ACIDS

L-ARGININE: Plays a role in sperm motility. It is also found in seminal fluids.

L-CYSTEINE, L-METHIONINE: Sulphur containing amino acids.

Here is a formula that is available in the marketplace today that would be beneficial for providing most of the nutritional support for the female:

Vitamin A (Fish Liver Oil)
Vitamin C (With Rose Hips)
Vitamin E (D-Alpha Tocopheryl)
Vitamin B1
Pantothenic Acid
Niacin
Folic Acid
Unsaturated Fatty Acids
Zinc (Amino Acid Chelate)
Ginseng Root
Damiana
Licorice Root
False Unicorn
Red Raspberry
Gotu Kola
Sarsaparilla
Wild Yam Root
Capsicum
Cloves
Yohimbe

Here is how the nutrients work in the body:

VITAMINS

VITAMINS A, C, E AND ZINC: (See Above)
PANTOTHENIC ACID: Essential in cellular metabolism.
NIACIN: Essential for the synthesis of sex hormones.

HERBS

GINSENG, DAMIANA & GOTU KOLA: Known as sexual rejuvenators.
LICORICE ROOT & WILD YAM ROOT: These herbs have estrogen producing characteristics.
FALSE UNICORN: Known to strengthen female uterine walls.
SARSAPARILLA: Contains hormone like substances and is valuable in glandular strengthening formulas.

Knowing that you can find these nutrients in a formula that will deliver most of the prime ingredients, here is how I recommend to take them: 1 or 2 tablets each meal. 3 each meal prior to and during fertility cycle.

PSYCHOLOGICAL CONSIDERATIONS

These possible combinations could prove to be very effective if:

1. The psychological considerations are openly discussed and resolved.

2. Prior to the effort of conception, an increase of these possible combinations is instituted, i.e. a week before, double or even triple the suggestions above. During the week, double the formula.

Gall Stones

Gall stones are the result of too much fried food and a diet high in cholestrol. The stones that are formed really have a cholesterol type base. Because of this type of structure they can easily be dissolved by using the following technique, (which I might add has worked time and time again):

Take 3 tablespoons of cold pressed olive oil and one (1) teaspoon of fresh squeezed lemon juice and then wait for 15 minutes.

AND REPEAT THE PROCESS

Take 3 tablespoons of cold pressed olive oil and one (1) teaspoon of fresh squeezed lemon juice and then wait for 15 minutes.

Continue this process untill you have consumed 6 to 9 oz. of olive oil. Then eat a large salad.

This entire project should be started on an empty stomach first thing in the morning. If you should happen to throw up, simply rinse out your mouth and continue.

The very first bowel movement that you have will contain gall stones. In all the years that I have been suggesting this approach I have never heard of one problem other than the taste of the olive oil.

Glaucoma

Glaucoma is a disease of the eyes marked by increased pressure within the eyeball that soon damages the optic nerve. Currently it affects over two million Americans. If detected early on, it can be nutritionally remedied or sometimes cured by laser surgery.

THOSE AT RISK

The most common type of glaucoma is the open-angle kind. It's without symptoms in the earliest stages, producing an entirely painless increase in eyeball pressure. Side or peripheral vision can be affected, but only slowly. Those at greatest risk are: (A) Anyone with a family history of this disease; (B) Blacks; (C) The severely nearsighted; (D) Diabetics; (E) Elderly over 65; and (F) Anyone on hypertension drugs or cortisone.

TREATMENT

"Glaucoma can't be cured, but can be controlled," states author John Kirschmann in his best-seller, *Nutrition Almanic* (McGraw-Hill, 1979). He recommends "a diet rich in vitamin A for those affected." Furthermore, he includes B-complex, especially inositol.

The Journal of Holistic Medicine (Fall/Winter, 1981) reported that vitamin C can help glaucoma by increasing osmotic pressure in the blood, which in turn pulls fluid out of the eyeball. Doctors in Rome found a dramatic drop in the eye pressures of all their glaucoma patients within two hours after a single dose of vitamin C was used. An Ohio optometrist found substantial drops in eye pressure and improved vision in his glaucoma patients when they took 500 mg. of C morning and evening for up to four months (*Optometric Monthly* August, 1983).

Here is a formula that is available in the marketplace today that would be beneficial for providing most of the nutritional support for this condition:

VITAMIN A (fish liver oil)	SELENIUM
VITAMIN D (fish liver oil)	ZINC
VITAMIN E (d alpha tocopherol)	PAPAYOTIN
VITAMIN B1 (Thiamine)	BROMELIN
VITAMIN B2 (Riboflavin)	PANCREATIN
VITAMIN B6 (Pyridoxine)	L-GLYCINE
VITAMIN B12 (Cobalamin)	L-GLUTAMINE
INOSITOL	L-ARGININE
FOLIC ACID (Folacin)	L-CYSTEINE HCL
NIACIN (Nicotinic Acid)	L-GLUTATHIONE
PANTOTHENIC ACID	EYEBRIGHT
VITAMIN C (Ascorbic Acid)	CHICKWEED
BIOFLAVONOID (Vitamin P)	CARDAMON
CALCIUM (Amino Acid Chelate)	GINGER
MAGNESIUM	RED RASPBERRY LEAVES

Here are the nutrients and why they help:

VITAMINS

VITAMIN A: Formation of rich blood, maintenance of good eye-sight. Essential in the formation of visual purple, a substance in the eye which is necessary for proper night vision.

VITAMIN E: Vitamin E is an antioxidant. As a diuretic, vitamin E helps lower elevated blood pressure. Protects against the damaging effects of many environmental poisons in the air, water and food.

VITAMIN B1 (Thiamine): Thiamine, essential for proper nerve function.

VITAMIN B2 (Riboflavin): Cataract can easily be produced in laboratory animals by depriving them of riboflavin. So diets deficient in vitamin C can produce scurvy. These same diets can also produce cataracts. A diet low in protein has also been linked to this eye disorder. A deficiency of riboflavin can cause anemia, visual fatigue, a "sandy" feeling of the eyes, inability to endure bright lights. Seborrhea, a scaly skin disease, is also a symptom of riboflavin deficiency.

VITAMIN B6 (Pyridoxine): That getting enough of the B vitamin would help to prevent raised cholesterol levels. Those patients with hardening of the arteries were found to have very low levels of pyridoxine in their blood. Pyridoxine has been found to be an anti-coagulant.

VITAMIN B12: Helps iron function better, aids folic acid in the synthesis of choline. Helps the placement of vitamin A into body tissues by aiding carotene absorption or vitamin A conversion. It has been used with some success in treating Glaucoma, treating this condition by injecting vitamin B12. A Japanese physician has confirmed the Russian findings by giving one milligram of vitamin B12.

INOSITOL: Inositol is closely related in function to the B vitamins choline and biotin.

VITAMIN B3 (Niacin): Niacin appears to reduce the level of cholesterol in the blood. The large doses of niacin brought about a reduction in cholesterol without any change in diet. It also provides more blood to all areas of the body.

VITAMIN C (Ascorbic Acid): protects thiamine, riboflavin, folic acid, pantothenic acid, and vitamin A and E against oxidation.

BIOFLAVONOID (Vitamin P): The components of the bioflavonoid are citrin, hesperidin, rutin, flavones, and flavonals. Essential for the proper absorption and use of vitamin C.

PANTOTHENIC ACID (B5): Essential constituent of coenzyme A, which forms active acetate and, as such, acts as an activating agent in metabolism.

MINERALS

CALCIUM: Calcium assists in the process of blood clotting and helps prevent the accumulation of too much acid or too much alkali in the blood.

MAGNESIUM: Magnesium activates more enzymes in the body than any other mineral.

ZINC: The vascular coating of the eye contains more zinc than any other part of the body. Zinc is essential for the treatment of arteriosclerosis. Zinc is essential, it seems, to "mobilize" vitamin A from the liver, so that it can perform its usual bodily functions.

SELENIUM: Is a natural antioxidant and appears to preserve elasticity of tissue by delaying oxidation of polyunsaturated fatty acids.

AMINO ACIDS

L-GLUTAMINE: Can readily cross the blood-barrier into the brain where it is quickly converted into glutamic acid. Serves primarily as a fuel for the brain which also keeps excess amounts of ammonia from damaging the brain.

L-CYSTEINE HCL: Involved in antibody production.

L-GLUTATHIONE: Protects the lens metabolism by preserving the physicochemical equilibrium of lens proteins, maintains the molecular integrity of the lens fiber membranes, protects membranes and organelles from oxidation.

HERBS

EYEBRIGHT: Sore and/or inflamed eyes.

CHICKWEED: Hemorrhoids, eye infections, (glaucoma, cataracts), blood diseases (leukemia, tetanus), and eczema.

RED RASPBERRY LEAVES: Astringent on the eyes (reducing mucous in them), hyperglycemia (abnormal amounts of glucose in the blood), cataracts that may be related to it.

SPECIAL DIETARY CONSIDERATIONS

ELIMINATE stimulants such as coffee or tea, excessive fluid intake whether juice, water or milk. Avoid emotional stress and upheavals. Also long movies, excessive TV watching and reading. Avoid smoking and using sunglasses.

INCREASE raw fresh fruits and vegetables. Specifics are Megadoses of vitamin C, rutin, vitamin A and choline.

DRINK lemon, grapefruit, orange, carrot, red beettop juice.

Goiter

See THYROID : PROGRAM M-THYR

High Blood Pressure

PROGRAM M-HE/P

HIGH BLOOD PRESSURE or HYPERTENSION as it is called by the medical community, is the result of today's lifestyle. We live in a fast paced and anxiety filled world in which we can easily become stressed to the point of hypertension.

Stress, tension and anxiety are not physical diseases although, they do cause them. Instead they are the results of mental attitudes about situations, how we look at things and how we react or feel about what we have seen.

Now, with that understanding in mind, we go beyond the medical approach of using diuretic type drugs to reduce the water content of the body. This is done in the belief that if the water content is reduced, the high blood pressure will also be reduced. To a point, this is true. But, to avoid a stroke or worse, more must be done to lower the blood pressure.

The following program will REDUCE HIGH BLOOD PRESSURE by ELIMINATION OF EXCESS WATER, MUSCULAR TENSION AND IT DILATES ARTERIES. IT ALSO EQUALIZES PRESSURE WITH CAYENNE.

Here is a formula that is available in the marketplace today that would be beneficial for providing most of the nutritional support for this condition:

Hawthorne Berries	Valerian Root
Apple Pectin	Hops
Garlic	Potassium (Amino Acid Complex)
Cayenne	Manganese (Amino Acid Chelate)
Vitamin B6 (Pyridoxine)	Calcium (Amino Acid Chelate)
Vitamin D (Fish Liver Oil)	L-Taurine (Amino Acid Free Form)
Black Cohosh	

Here is how the nutrients work in the body:

VITAMINS

VITAMIN B6: Aid in maintaining correct water balance in the blood and tissues.
VITAMIN D: Ensures the effectiveness of Calcium.

MINERALS

CALCIUM: Acts as a calmative on the muscles.
MANGANESE: Helps to nourish the nerves and the brain, kit is also used in the utilization of choline, a fat dissolving vitamin. Fats/cholesterol and triglycerides in the blood create circulation problems.

HERBS

APPLE PECTIN, GARLIC AND CAYENNE: All have the ability to equalize blood pressure.
HAWTHORNE BERRIES: Tone and strengthen the heart muscle.
VALERIAN ROOT AND HOPS: Calming herbs to the nervous system.

OTHER SYNERGISTIC NUTRIENTS

L-TAURINE: An amino acid is found in high amounts in the heart and central nervous system. Taurine aids in the metabolism of cholesterol and triglycerides.

Knowing that you can find these nutrients in a formula that will deliver most of the prime ingredients, here is how I recommend to take them: 1 tablet each meal.

SPECIAL DIETARY CONSIDERATIONS

ELIMINATE salt, artificial colors and flavors.
INCREASE intake of apples, watermelon, garlic, cucumbers, sesame seeds, pumpkin seeds.
DRINK caffeine free products, skullcap tea.

Hyperactivity

See STRESS AND TENSION (TRANQUILIZER) :
PROGRAM M-TRQ

Hypoglycemia

(Low Blood Sugar)

A specific for HYPOGLYCEMIA. Also good for a general uplift without the harsh effects of caffeine or ephedrine based herbs.

It is interesting to note how many people are constantly feeling tired and run down, even after a full nights sleep. In fact if you were to think about it you could probably think of some family members, friends and co-workers who complain of being tired all the time.

If you were really curious and started to ask them some simple questions like: do you always wake up tired after a full nights sleep; get drowsy after eating a heavy meal; feel like you need a nap around three in the afternoon; do you get cranky easily or emotionally upset or angry quickly? If these questions get more that a fifty percent positive response then you can bet that you are dealing with hypoglycemia. It's not as bad as it sounds.

Hypoglycemia is simply the medical term for low blood sugar. It is generally caused by poor dietary habits and / or stress.

It is interesting to note how many people try to deal with this problem by taking stimulants, such as B12 shots, the herbs Guarana, Ephedra(Ma Huang) or other type herbs that are high in caffeine. This approach is not the answer. It is only a form of relief without addressing the true cause.

One approach that will work, will help the person feel like a human being again lies within good nutrition and dietary changes.

Knowing how difficult it is to change eating habits, I have researched and found the nutritional elements that will help the body to correct hypoglycemia.

First let us examine how low blood sugar is created.

As we stated, one cause of low blood sugar is brought about by stress. When the body is subjected to stressful conditions, it depletes the adrenal glands. The adrenal glands are involved with blood sugar regulation. They "tell" the pancreas when to stop insulin production. Insulin, from the pancreas, is used to convert blood sugar from one form to another. When too much insulin is produced, then too much blood sugar is converted out of the "fuel" form and a drop in energy is experienced.

Now, if the adrenal glands are exhausted, depleted and unable to tell the pancreas to stop — you will have an energy let down. The way to avoid this is simple. Feed your adrenal glands, and energy will be there.

The following program improves communication between adrenal glands and pancreas for CONTROLLING SUGAR LEVELS in the blood. Works to nourish adrenal glands. Provides oxygen to brain and IMPROVES ENDURANCE.

Here is a formula that is available in the marketplace today that would be beneficial for providing most of the nutritional support for this condition:

Vitamin B12 (Cyanocobalamin)   Siberian Ginseng
Folic Acid   Gotu Kola
Pantothenic Acid   Licorice
Aspartic Acid (An Amino Acid)

Here is how the nutrients work in the body:

VITAMINS

PANTOTHENIC ACID: Provides nourishment to the adrenal glands. The adrenal glands work with the pancreas in maintaining proper blood sugar levels. This helps in keeping the energy levels up.
VITAMIN B12: Has been used by the medical profession for years to provide energy to tired and run down individuals.
FOLIC ACID: Works in conjunction with B12 to insure that anemia is corrected and / or prevented.

HERBS

LICORICE: Also nourishes the adrenal glands.
SIBERIAN GINSENG: Has been used for centuries as a tonic and is highly invigorating.
GOTU KOLA: Feeds and stimulates the mind as well as the body. It creates alertness.

OTHER SYNERGISTIC NUTRIENTS

ASPARTIC ACID: Helps in increasing stamina and endurance as well as resistance to fatigue.

Knowing that you can find these nutrients in a formula that will deliver most of the prime ingredients, here is how I recommend to take them: 1 tablet each meal for the first 4 days, then 1 in the morning, and 1 in the afternoon, if needed or 2 as desired or needed.

SPECIAL DIETARY CONSIDERATIONS

ELIMINATE sugar, salt, white flour products, fried foods, high amounts of protein.
INCREASE fresh and raw vegetables — parsley, cucumbers, beets, spinach, dark leafy green vegetables: endive, lettuce. Fruits — not more than 1 at a time.
DRINK ginseng tea, licorice tea.

Immune Boosting

Designed to provide the full range of IMMUNE BOOSTING nutrients currently available. Its best use is as a preventative maintenance program. NOTE: When illness is present this formula could be used with formula M-CO, which should always be your first choice to directly fight infection.

In today's world of AIDS and other degenerative diseases we are faced with the fact that our bodies especially our immune systems are no longer able to defend us. There seems to have been a weakening of that system. Why is that so?

There are always two sides to every story. For the purpose of our discussion we will touch on two aspects that are instrumental in weakening the immune system.

First we need to recall the latest research that is taking place in regards to stress. It is being demonstrated and proven that stress adversely affects the immune system.

Stress taxes the adrenal glands which secrete hormones that carry messages to the other glands on how and/or what to perform or manufacture. All of the glands of the body are tied together in a complicated system. Each and every aspect of life within the body is dependent on each other. This is why it is so important to maintain a proper nutritional balance within. In this way you are providing the system with the needed ingredients to function correctly and thus provide optimum health. It also eliminates the opportunity for disease to take hold.

It appears that stress depletes nutrients that are vital to the health of the immune system. When this happens the immune system does not perform at efficient levels and illness becomes more prevalent.

The inability of the immune system to destroy invaders sets up a condition in the body that allows invaders to take hold, and we are infected with some sort of germ.

At the same time another situation can take place. It may be the cause for all of the auto-immune diseases. Here is what happens; the bacteria that surrounds us all the time, on our skin, in the air and on the food we eat, enters into our bodies. Since the immune system is not strong enough to attack and destroy all of the invaders some of them have the time, and the ability to adapt to the "new" environment, our blood stream. While in the blood stream they are able to enter into healthy cells and become a part of that cell. This creates a condition where the antibodies do not know who to attack. The invaders are now a part of the cells that the body has always recognized as its own. Now these mutated cells have an opportunity to multiply. The result is a body full of "sick" cells. Cells that have the ability to destroy the body. Arthritis is thought to be one such condition, an auto-immune disease.

AIDS may very well be another one of these types of diseases. Which brings us back to the true cause, a very weakened immune system.

Now we have said that stress is one of the culprits responsible for this condition and has to be dealt with. This is more difficult to correct than the other cause that we mentioned, nutritional deficiencies.

Poor nutrition has been the cause of countless diseases throughout time. Scurvy, rickets,and pellagra are just a few examples.

Nutrition, or more correctly, nutrients are the building materials of the human body. They are the building blocks, cement, wood and nails of life — nothing is created within the human body without an adequate supply of these nutrients. Nor is any system able to maintain itself without the proper nutrients in the correct amounts.

When you try to maintain good health (strong immune system) and you don't have all the right nutrients or proper amounts you can not have a sound and healthy immune system.

So, the two causes of a weak and ineffective immune system are stress and poor nutrition. Stress is a perception and attitude problem that requires a particular form of adjustments. Nutrition is a dietary and supplementation adjustment.

In regards to the dietary changes the most obvious would be to include more fresh fruits and raw vegetables. Increasing garlic, onions, celery, watercress and carrots would be especially helpful. Decreasing all fried and fatty foods along with curtailing the amount of meat, fish and fowl that you eat would also be wise.

Here is a formula that is available in the marketplace today that would be beneficial for providing most of the nutritional support for this condition:

Beta Carotene (pro vitamin A)	Co Q10
Vitamin E	S.O.D.(superoxide dismutase)
Vitamin B1	Germanium Sesquioxide
Vitamin B2	Echinacea
Vitamin B6	Astragalus
Vitamin C	Rei-Shi mushroom
Choline	Codonopis
Inositol	White Astractylodes
Folic Acid	Schizandra Berries
Pantothenic Acid	Ligustrum Berries
Magnesium	Watercress
Selenium	Shiitake mushroom
Zinc	Juniper Berries
L-Cysteine	

Here is how the nutrients work in the body:

VITAMINS

VITAMIN E: Prevents saturated fatty acids and vitamin A from breaking down and combining with other substances that may become harmful to the body. Vitamin B complex and ascorbic acid are also protected against oxidation when Vitamin E is present in the digestive tract.

PANTOTHENIC ACID: Stimulates the adrenal glands and increases production of cortisone and other adrenal hormones. Can improve the body's ability to withstand stressful conditions.

VITAMIN B2: Protection of cellular respiration.

VITAMIN B6: Must be present for the production of antibodies and red blood cells. Improves T-cell levels and mitogen stimulation.

CHOLINE: Essential for the health of the liver and kidneys. Essential for the health of the myelin sheaths of the nerves; the myelin sheaths are the principal component of the nerve fibers. In the transmission of the nerve impulses.

PANTOTHENIC ACID: Has been demonstrated to enhance the activity of macrophage and natural killer cells in the body. Necessary for antibody production, which is part of the humoral branch of the immune system.

FOLIC ACID: Is involved in the formation of white blood cells and lymphocytes, the front line soldiers of the immune system.

VITAMIN C: Fights bacterial infections and reduces the effects on the body of some allergy-producing substances.

MINERALS

MAGNESIUM: Activates more enzymes in the body than any other mineral. Lack of magnesium may be involved as one of the causes of one kind of leukemia, or cancer of the blood.

SELENIUM: Appears to prevent certain kinds of cancer.

GERMANIUM: Induces interferon to increase germanium-oxygen combination has been found to suppress tumor growth in both animals and humans.

ZINC: Is essential, it seems, to "mobilize" vitamin A from the liver, so that it can perform its usual bodily functions. Protects the immune system and supports the T-cells. When zinc intake is decreased, the thymus atrophies.

HERBS

ECHINACEA: Induces living cells to excrete more of the interferon, which the cells already manufacture. Destroys the germs of infection directly, bolsters the body's defenses by magnifying the white blood cell count. Echinacin, the active constituent of Echinacea, interferon-like activity. It protects cells against virus related diseases, such as herpes, influenza, canker sores, etc. Ability to stimulate T-cell activity.

ASTRAGALUS: Increases in phagocytose, interferon and cancer survival.

LIGUSTRUM: Increases in WBC's in cancer patients.

GANODERMA: Also called the rei-shi mushroom in Japan, increases phagocytosis, macrophage, and cell mediated immunity; suppresses tumor growth in mice.

WHITE ASTRACTYLODES: Increases WBC's and phagocytosis.

CODONOPIS: Increases phagocytosis, red blood cells, and T-cell transformation.

OTHER SYNERGISTIC NUTRIENTS

S.O.D. (superoxide dismutase): Is essentially known for its ability to eliminate free radicals. In this particular formula we are not focusing on free radical elimination but it is an integral part of immune boosting. Free radicals are known to cause cancer and other degenerative diseases. Since it is our goal to strengthen the immune system, it pays to reduce the causative factors that would cause it to work overtime.

BETA CAROTENE: Is converted into Vitamin A in the body. As vitamin A it feeds and strengthens the thymus gland, which is responsible for how the body responds to infections.

L-CYSTEINE: Is involved in antibody production.

Knowing that you can find these nutrients in a formula that will deliver most of the prime ingredients, here is how I recommend to take them: 1 or 2 tablets in the morning; 1 or 2 tablets in the evening.

SPECIAL DIETARY CONSIDERATIONS

ELIMINATE all artificial additives and caffeine. All white flour products, and sugar. Fried foods and anything else that slows down or taxes the workings of the body.

INCREASE fresh and raw fruits and vegetable especially garlic, onions, watercress, and carrots. Sprouts would also be excellent to bring into the diet.

DRINK clean pure distilled water. Echinacea tea.

Impotence

An excellent approach to IMPOTENCE and SEXUAL RE-JUVENATION.

In today's high stressed world, we often find ourselves unable to perform in life as we once did. This applies to all aspects of life.

One of the most frustrating areas is sexual expression, with the result being an inability to perform.

The causes go beyond simple stress. In some instances there is poor circulation. Others deal with diabetes, some with side effects from medication and some suffer from psychological causes.

There is an herb that has been in use for centuries to assist man in maintaining his "nature". This herb is called Yohimbe, the inner bark of the tropical West African tree Corynanthe Yohimbe. The material contains several indole-based alkaloids, of which yohimbine is the most prominent. It causes increased vasodilation and peripheral blood flow in combination with stimulation of the spinal ganglia which controls the corpus spongiosum (erectile tissue). This action produces erections in the male. Other pleasurable effects are warm spinal shivers, which is especially enjoyable during coitus and orgasm (bodies feel like they are melting into one another), psychic stimulations, mild perceptual changes without hallucination and heightening of emotional and sexual feeling. Effects last about two hours.

Yohimbine is also a mild serotonin inhibitor. It has been found that when larger than normal amounts of serotonin are produced in the body, blood pressure, nervousness, depression and exhaustion are increased. There is a possibility that some forms of impotence are not psychologically based or due to any waning of one's glandular manhood, but may simply be the result of increased serotonin levels in the brain. Conversely, substances which inhibit serotonin are likely to have an apparent aphrodisiacal influence. This response, however, is in fact the natural sex chemistry of the body being liberated pharmaceutically from the blockage of the serotonin.

Normally there are no undesirable after-effects. Individuals with sensitive stomachs may experience some queasiness or mild nausea for a few minutes shortly after drinking the tea. It is best to sip it slowly. Yohimbe should not be used by persons suffering from blood pressure disorders, diabetes, hypoglycemia, or active ailments or injury of kidneys liver or heart. It is a brief-acting monoamine oxidase inhibitor and should not be used by persons under the influence of alcohol, amphetamines (even diet pills), antihistamines, narcotics and certain tranquilizers.

Yohimbe works directly on the sex center of the brain as well as other organs. In the brain it inhibits serotonin, which we stated earlier increases blood pressure, exhaustion and feelings of depression.

Yohimbe has been found to be very effective in re-establishing a sexual relationship. It can be taken by both men and women.

Works to stimulate sexual center in brain and direct stimulation upon sex organ. NOTE: Psychological counseling is highly recommended as most impotence problems arise from feeling of inadequacy and often reinforced through assertive / successful mate.

Here is a formula that is available in the marketplace today that would be beneficial for providing most of the nutritional support for this condition:

Yohimbe	Dong Quai
Damiana	Zinc (Amino Acid Chelate)
Siberian Ginseng	Vitamin E (D-Alpha tocopherol)

Here is how these nutrients work in the body:

HERBS

YOHIMBE BARK: Contains yohimbine, a strong sexual stimulant. Also used as a general tonic. Can be used by women.

SIBERIAN GINSENG, DONG QUAI, AND DAMIANA: Are all famous for their "aphrodisiac" type properties.

MINERALS

ZINC (amino acid chelate): Nourishes the prostate gland as well as being important in sperm production.

Knowing that you can find these nutrients in a formula that will deliver most of the prime ingredients, here is how I recommend to take them: 1 to 3 (possibly 4) capsules taken 1 or 2 hours before intercourse. It may be best to start with 3 capsules and adjust accordingly.

SPECIAL DIETARY CONSIDERATIONS

ELIMINATE alcohol. It makes the heart speed up when taken within 1½ hours of taking Yohimbe.

Intestinal Cleansing

Excellent for CLEANING OUT THE INTESTINAL TRACT. Tones and nourishes as it cleans.

The fitness of the intestinal tract cannot be over emphasized. Like the importance of the other cleansing organs, it is imperative to excellent health that this particular system be free of mucus and other factors that would have a tendency to clog the villi.

The villi, which looks like little fingers, have little openings between them from where they hang in the intestines. This opening is where the nutrients are absorbed into the blood stream for distribution to all parts of the body. If the villi are clogged for any reason then the amount of nutrients that should be entering into the blood, for food for the cells, is diminished. In addition to decreased nourishment there is the fact that the body makes the effort to absorb what it can through the villi openings. The body does not know what it is bringing into the blood stream, it only knows that it should be absorbing anything that is available to it. With this in mind it becomes important to remove all the harmful pollutants that are in the intestines as quick as possible. The sooner that this is done the quicker the body can respond to the nutrients that are available to it.

Here is a formula that is available in the marketplace today that would be beneficial for providing most of the nutritional support for this condition:

Psyllium Husks	Comfrey
Flax Seeds	Pepsin
Rice Bran	Pumpkin Seed
Perch Bark	Garlic
Apple Pectin	Dandelion Root
Clay (Montmorillonite)	Butternut Bark
Slippery Elm	Cascara Sagrada
Marshmallow Root	

Here is how these herbs work in the body:

SLIPPERY ELM BARK: Effective, both internally and externally, against sore and inflamed mucous membranes.

PUMPKIN SEED: Its main use continues to be as an anthelmintic (parasitic killer).

BUTTERNUT ROOT BARK: For its mild laxative property.

GARLIC: One mg of its major constituent, allicin, is estimated to equal 15 standard units of penicillin.

MARSHMALLOW ROOT: Soothes mucous membranes. Used internally to treat inflammation and mucosal afflictions.

CASCARA SAGRADA: An aid in restoring the natural tone of the colon. Used in smaller amounts in folk medicine to treat liver disorders and gallstones. Herb to treat jaundice and other hepatic conditions.

COMFREY ROOT, MARSHMALLOW ROOT AND SLIPPERY ELM BARK: Are all mucilaginous in quality. Because of their slick adhesiveness, they coat the lower bowels with a nutritious substance that strengthens as well as heals.

Knowing that you can find these herbs in a formula that will deliver most of the prime ingredients, here is how I recommend to take them: 2 or 3 at each meal and 3 before bed.

Kidney Cleansing _____

Great for removing KIDNEY GRAVEL and STONES. Also effective as a stimulator and general cleanser for the kidneys.

The reason we are going to work on the kidneys next is because they have been filtering the blood stream and extracting the toxins for elimination. There is the possibility that gravel and other forms of "pollution" have been accumulating in the kidneys. There is also the consideration that they have been working "overtime" to keep the blood stream free from re-absorbing the toxins made water soluble by the liver.

Here is a formula that is available in the marketplace today that would be beneficial for providing most of the nutritional support for this condition:

Celery Seed   Buchu Leaf
Hydrangea   Uva Ursi Leaves
Parsley   Magnesium (Amino Acid Chelate)
Juniper Berries   Bromelin (Pineapple Enzyme)
Queen of the Meadow   Vitamin D (Fish Liver Oil)

Here is how these nutrients work in the body:

HERBS

HYDRANGEA: Used for bladder and kidney disorders, including stones, inflammation, and backache from kidney trouble.
CELERY SEED: Diuretic activity.
JUNIPER BERRY: Directly on the kidneys. High volatile oil content (especially terpinol). Its primary application is as a diuretic.
UVA URSI LEAVES: Disinfectant properties, urinary antiseptic, chronic cystitis or bladder inflammation, nephritis, or kidney inflammation, and kidney stones, diabetes.
BUCHU LEAF: Urinary disinfectant, mildly diuretic. Mainly for diseases of the kidney, urinary tract and prostate.
QUEEN OF THE MEADOW: Primarily as a diuretic (for which reason it is often called gravel root), especially where uric acid levels are high.

OTHER SYNERGISTIC NUTRIENTS

MAGNESIUM: Lack of magnesium can lead to calcium deposits in muscles, the heart, and kidneys.

Knowing that you can find these nutrients in a formula that will deliver most of the prime ingredients, here is how I recommend to take them: 1 or 2 tablets each meal.

SPECIAL DIETARY CONSIDERATIONS

ELIMINATE vegetables with large quantities of oxalic acid, such as spinach and rhubarb, chocolate and cocoa.

INCREASE garlic, potatoes, asparagus, parsley, horseradish, watercress, cucumber and celery. Best fruits are papaya, bananas and watermelon is excellent. Also include goat's milk, homemade cottage cheese, unfiltered honey and brown rice.

DRINK watermelon, cucumber and celery juice. Small amounts of juice from horseradish, watercress and garlic added to carrot juice. Cranberry juice.

Kidney Stones

See KIDNEY CLEANSER : M-RE / F

Laxative

The goal here is to provide a gentle, but effective laxative that will not cramp the bowels.

The need for a laxative is because constipation exists due to the body's inability to evacuate fecal matter properly.

Constipation is generally caused by poor choices of foods. Most of the American diet consist of foods that have been so processed that the fiber content has been removed. It is the fiber that acts as a "broom" sweeping through the alimentary canal that keeps the "house" clean.

Another consideration is the fact that this same processing eliminates most of the nutrients, including minerals, which are so important for the peristaltic action of the large intestines.

Here is a formula that is available in the marketplace today that would be a gentle laxative:

Butternut Bark	Plantain Leaves & Seeds	Senna	Licorice
Flax Seed	Cascara Sagrada	Prunes	Buckthorn Bark

Here is how these nutrients work in the body:

BUTTERNUT ROOT BARK, BUCKTHORN BARK, SENNA: Primarily known for their mild laxative properties.

FLAX SEED, PLANTAIN LEAVES & SEEDS: These provide "pushing and scraping" benefits.

CASCARA SAGRADA: An aid in restoring the natural tone of the colon. Used in smaller amounts in folk medicine to treat liver disorders and gallstones.

Knowing that you can find these nutrients in a formula that will deliver most of the prime ingredients, here is how I recommend to take them: 2 or 3 before bed with plenty of clean water.

SPECIAL DIETARY CONSIDERATIONS

ELIMINATE all refined and processed foods. Avoid salt, sugar and white flour, coffee, tea and alcohol.

INCREASE high residue vegetables and fruits; raw and cooked, whole grains, seeds and nuts. Also sprouted seeds. Foods to be used regularly: homemade sauerkraut, sesame seeds, soaked prunes and dried figs. Morning and evening: yogurt, kefir or other soured milks; honey, natural, unfiltered. Include alfalfa and mung beans, raw fruits, especially apples and vegetables. And 2 tbsp. of cold pressed olive, sesame, safflower daily.

DRINK plenty of juices: spinach, watercress, nettles, (add small amounts of garlic and yellow onions to vegetable juices). Black radish and dandelion added to milder juices of carrots, cucumber, and celery. Also included are fruit juices: apple and lemon.

Leg Aches

See OSTEOPOROSIS : PROGRAM M-OS.

Liver Cleansing
PROGRAM M-HEP/F

An effective LIVER DETOXIFIER. Great for reducing fatty deposits. Increases liver efficiency.

When the liver is being cleansed it functions better which help the digestive system to perform more efficiently. This also helps in the elimination of toxic material from the body.

The liver is also tied into the kidneys by processing the toxins into water disposable products. That way the kidneys can work with the material to get it out of the body.

Here is a formula that is available in the marketplace today that would be beneficial for providing most of the nutritional support for this condition:

Lecithin
Chickweed
Dandelion Root
Chaparral

Stillingia Root
Fumitory
Beet Root
Chicory Root

Here is how these nutrients work in the body:

HERBS

CHICKWEED: Antibiotic properties.

DANDELION ROOT: Stimulates liver activity, encouraging the elimination of toxins in the blood. It stimulates the flow of bile and excretion of urea. Successfully treats hepatitis, swelling of the liver, jaundice and dyspepsia with deficient bile secretion.

CHAPARRAL: Inhibits several strains of bacteria, molds and other pathogens.

STILLINGIA ROOT: Glandular activator(especially liver). Aids skin, urinary and respiratory systems. Used for obstinate skin problems and especially valuable as an internal cleansing agent to rid the system of toxic drugs.

CHICORY ROOT: Has properties very similar to dandelion. Often used for jaundice and spleen problems. Promotes the production of bile, the release of gallstones, and the elimination of excessive internal mucus.

FUMITORY: Used primarily for liver and gallbladder problems. Also in stomach and skin disorders.

VITAMIN

LECITHIN: Keeps cholesterol more soluble, detoxifies the liver, and increases resistance to disease by helping the thymus gland carry out its functions.

Knowing that you can find these nutrients in a formula that will deliver most of the prime ingredients, here is how I recommend to take them: 1 or 2 tablets at each meal.

SPECIAL DIETARY CONSIDERATIONS

ELIMINATE large meals, fats, oils, processed canned and refined foods. Avoid chemical additives, synthetic vitamins, drugs, salt, spices, sugar, alcohol.

INCREASE brewer's yeast, raw goat's milk, raw cottage cheese, sprouted seeds and grains, raw nuts, especially almonds and sesame seed butter (Tahini). Also include red beets, endive, artichoke, cucumber, garlic and lemon.

DRINK red beet juice, lemon juice, papaya juice, grape juice. Radish, black radish and dandelion juice added in small amounts to beet juice.

Low Blood Sugar _____

See HYPOGLYCEMIA : PROGRAM M-PE / U

Have you ever started to introduce a friend or colleague to one another and you couldn't recall their names? How about looking at a phone number and by the time you looked back at the dial or push buttons you don't recall the last two or three digits?

These are everyday occurrences that make you feel very uncomfortable. But you can take heart, for these are "normal" situations according to the experts. Even though the "experts" tell us that a little bit of forgetfulness is common it does not help to alleviate the fear that something is wrong with you. You immediately think that you have Alzheimer's disease.

The thought of getting Alzheimer's disease is enough to scare you into taking action in a preventative way if only you really knew what to do. In order to form a plan of action that would help to protect you from this dreaded disease you need to understand exactly what this disease is all about. Unfortunately there isn't too much medical knowledge available. Why is this so?

Doctors, by the very nature of their healing system, refuse to see diseases as the result of poor nutrition, or that they may be caused by the "AMERICAN DIET". It lies within a protective belief system. If they were to accept that the human body is the result of what goes into it, then by changing the input would change the results. This would also validate what the health food people say: "most diseases can be healed or controlled and/or prevented with good nutrition."

Those of us in the natural healing arts know that Alzheimer's is a disease that is the result of poor nutrition and bad circulation. Let's first look at the circulation aspect.

The blood is the life line of the body. It feeds each and every cell within the entire system. When it comes to the brain, it can only "present" the nutrients that the brain requires because blood does not enter into the brain matter. There is a protective "envelope" called the "blood barrier". Its purpose is to prevent blood from passing into the brain. It does accept the nutrients that the brain needs and passes those through so that the brain can feed and nourish itself.

Now if the blood is thick with cholesterol and triglycerides then the amount of "nutrient rich" blood is severely restricted and the amount that passes by the "barrier" becomes even less. When this happens you can begin to imagine how little of the available nutrients are able to feed the brain. It is no wonder that the brain is starving to death, dying a little bit each day. This may be the main reason that people begin to forget.

This brings us to the next area of concern, memory or your ability to recall information when you need it. The mind works because of neurotransmitters.

Neurotransmitters are nutrients that act as "switches" in the brain. They allow the electrical nerve impulses to pass, they permit ALL of the functions of the body to take place in proper sequence. You can begin to imagine what can take place when the brain does not have an adequate amount of neurotransmitters, or the nutrients available to make them. You would have "shorts". In electrical terms you would have a power failure or a device would not work properly and may even burn up. The brain is confronted with the same kind of situation. It does not make the right or complete connections and therefore there is a "short". The mind goes blank or it begins to plug in to an old, disconnected, memory, or circuit. We call this confusion, disorientation, lapse of memory, senility, and of course Alzheimer's disease. There is a way to fortify the brain with the proper amount of nutrients necessary to create neurotransmitters.

Here is a formula that is available in the marketplace today that would be beneficial for providing most of the nutritional support for this condition:

VITAMIN E (d alpha tocopherol)
VITAMIN F (unsaturated fatty acids)
VITAMIN B1 (Thiamine)
VITAMIN B6 (Pyridoxine)
CHOLINE (Choline bitartrate)
INOSITOL
FOLIC ACID (Folacin)
NIACIN (Nicotinic Acid)
NIACINAMIDE
PANTOTHENIC ACID
PABA (Para Aminobenzoic Acid)
MAGNESIUM (Amino acid chelate)
MANGANESE (Amino acid chelate)
POTASSIUM (Amino acid complex)
SELENIUM (Amino acid chelate)
ZINC (Amino acid chelate)
S.O.D. (SuperOxide Dismutase)
GOTU KOLA
MADAGASCAR PERIWINKLE
L-GLUTAMINE (Free form amino acid)
L-METHIONINE (Free form amino acid)
L-TYROSINE (Free form amino acid)
L-TAURINE (Free form amino acid)
L-GLUTATHIONE (Free form amino acid)
LECITHIN
ACETYLCHOLINE
PHOSPHATIDYL CHOLINE
DMAE (Dimethyl amino ethanol)

Here are the nutrients and why they help:

VITAMINS

VITAMIN E: Causes dilation of the blood vessels, permitting a fuller flow of blood.

VITAMIN F (UNSATURATED FATTY ACIDS (UFA)): Makes it easier for oxygen to be transported by the bloodstream. Helps perform a vital function in breaking up cholesterol deposited on arterial walls.

VITAMIN B1 (THIAMINE): Beneficial effect on mental attitude and a healthy nervous system. Linked with improving individual learning capability.

VITAMIN B6: Promotes the normal functioning of the nervous and musculoskeletal systems.

CHOLINE: Is known as a fat burner and works to dissolve fats in the blood stream.

INOSITOL: Co-functions with choline as a fat burner.

FOLIC ACID: Essential for mental and emotional health.

NIACIN, NIACINAMIDE: Improving circulation and reducing the cholesterol level in the blood. Niacin is important for improving memory.

PANTOTHENIC ACID: Important for healthy skin and nerves and vital in cellular metabolism.

MINERALS

MAGNESIUM: Magnesium plays an important role in neuromuscular contractions.

MANGANESE: Helps nourish the nerves and brain. Aids in the utilization of choline.

POTASSIUM: Unites with phosphorus to send oxygen to the brain and also functions with calcium in the regulation of neuromuscular activity.

SELENIUM: A natural antioxidant and appears to preserve elasticity of tissue by delaying oxidation of polyunsaturated fatty acids.

ZINC: May be involved in binding a certain substance in a certain part of the brain so that it is there to perform its function. That part of brain contains considerable amount of zinc.

S.O.D. (superoxide dismutase): Is essentially known for its ability to eliminate free radicals.

HERBS

GOTU KOLA: Specifically to improve memory and longevity. Excellent oxygen carrier.

MADAGASCAR PERIWINKLE: Carries more oxygen to the brain than any other herb known.

AMINO ACIDS

GLUTAMIC ACID: The principal amino acid contributor to brain energy supplies.

L-GLUTAMINE: Can readily cross the blood-barrier into the brain where it is quickly converted into glutamic acid. Serves primarily as a fuel for the brain which also keeps excess amounts of ammonia from damaging the brain.

L-METHIONINE: Help nourish brain cells and help choline's effect in promoting thinking ability.

L-TYROSINE: Stimulates production of norepinephrine, the "alertness" brain chemical, has a role in sharpening learning, memory, and awareness, elevating mood and motivation.

LECITHIN: Excellent fat metabolizer.

ACETYLCHOLINE: Most important of the body's nuerotransmitters (brain chemicals that carry messages between neurons, facilitates learning, memory and intelligence). Key role is maximizing mental ability and prevents loss of memory in aging adults.

PHOSPHATIDYL CHOLINE: Acts as a fat metabolizer and is converted into acetylcholine, a neurotransmitter.

SPECIAL DIETARY CONSIDERATIONS

ELIMINATE all fried foods, fatty meats and most dairy products, white flour, sugar and salt. Also avoid hydrogenated fats and oils.

INCREASE the consumption of fresh fruits, anise, papaya, pineapple, apples, grapefruit, lemon juice. Also increase raw vegetables especially garlic, onions, artichokes, watercress, okra, dark leafy greens.

DRINK 2 tablespoons flax seed oil daily, dandelion tea, gotu kola tea, and/or ginseng tea.

EXCERCISE by laying on a slant board or in such a way as to have your head lower than your feet. This type of exercise will send additional blood to the brain.

Menopause

Especially for CHANGE OF LIFE, HOT FLASHES, hormonal balance.

There is probably nothing more discomforting that a woman's change of life. The "hot flashes", night sweats, mood changes, and other more subtle differences can be very annoying.

These changes are all brought about because of the decrease/lack of hormone production.

One specific hormone, Estrogen, is the one medical science focuses on when a woman goes through menopause. Estrogen is found in the ovaries and adrenals. In this way, estrogen production can still take place.

It is important to note two facts, first, that many women have had operations in which the ovaries have been removed. Secondly, the adrenals are considered the stress centers of the body. They are usually the first glands adversely affected by stress. And everybody deals with stress. So, what you have is a less than adequate production of estrogen.

It becomes necessary to work on three different nutritional levels.

1. If ovaries are present, nourish and rebuild, re-stimulate estrogen production.

2. Nourish and fortify adrenal glands.

3. If ovaries have been removed then we must bring in natural herbs that contain estrogenic properties.

With these understandings in mind the following nutrients will be helpful.

Here is a formula that is available in the marketplace today that would be beneficial for providing most of the nutritional support for this condition:

Wild Yam Root	Vitamin E (D-Alpha Tocopheryl)
Licorice	Pantothenic Acid
Unicorn Roots	Vitamin C (With Rose Hips)
Tangkuei	PABA (Para Aminobenzoic Acid)
Black Cohosh	Iodine (Kelp)
Passion Flower	Calcium (Amino Acid Chelate)

Here is how the nutrients work in the body:

VITAMINS

PANTOTHENIC ACID: Nourish the adrenal glands.

VITAMIN E: An anti-oxidant, helps prevent hormones produced in the adrenal glands from being oxidized.

VITAMIN C: Is found in large quantities within the adrenal glands and is needed in sex glands as aging takes place.

VITAMIN B6: Excellent for women who are suspectable to finger joint pain that often accompanies menopause.

MINERALS

IODINE: Nourishes the thyroid.
CALCIUM: In insufficient amounts cause a decrease in estrogen production.

HERBS

WILD YAM ROOT, BLACK COHOSH AND LICORICE: Have all been used to provide estrogen type properties to the body.
UNICORN ROOTS: Cleanse and strengthen ovaries.
TANGKUEI ALSO KNOWN AS DONG QUAI: Is considered one of the best herbs for females because it does so many different things within the reproduction system.

Knowing that you can find these nutrients in a formula that will deliver most of the prime ingredients, here is how I recommend to take them: three (3) tablets at each meal for the first day. Then take two (2) tablets at each meal for the next three days, then take 1 tablet at each meal.

Obesity

See WEIGHT LOSS: PROGRAM M-TRM
AND ALSO
WATER RETENTION: PROGRAM M-WA.

Osteoporosis

An efficient approach to OSTEOPOROSIS. Also beneficial for BACK-ACHES, LEG ACHES AND TOE CRAMPS.

The most interesting thing about osteoporosis or bone loss is — you lose more calcium throughout the night while you are sleeping than during the day when you are STANDING UP!

Based on that data some researchers suggest calcium supplements are better taken right before going to bed.

Another point to consider is that you need to have the right complimentary nutrients to insure that you will assimilate the calcium you take.

This program provides most COMPLETE AND ASSIMILABLE CALCIUM for bone, muscle, and nerve use. Calcium relieves cramps, backaches, poor sleep patterns, stress, tension.

Here is a formula that is available in the marketplace today that would be beneficial for providing most of the nutritional support for this condition:

Calcium (Amino Acid Chelate)
Magnesium (Amino Acid Chelate)
Phosphorus (Amino Acid Chelate)
Zinc (Amino Acid Chelate)
Vitamin D (Fish Liver Oil)
Vitamin A (Fish Liver Oil)
Vitamin C (Ascorbic Acid)
Betaine HCL
Alfalfa
Horsetail Grass

Here is how these nutrients work in the body:

MINERALS

CALCIUM, MAGNESIUM, ZINC & PHOSPHORUS: Essential for calcium assimilation.

HERBS

ALFALFA: Contain easily assimilative forms of calcium.
HORSETAIL GRASS: For silica.

OTHER SYNERGISTIC NUTRIENTS

VITAMIN D, BETAINE HCL: For calcium assimilation.

Knowing that you can find these nutrients in a formula that will deliver most of the prime ingredients, here is how I recommend to take them: 2 or 3 tablets 1/2 hour before retiring.

SPECIAL DIETARY CONSIDERATIONS

ELIMINATE fried and fatty foods.
INCREASE green leafy vegetables, sesame seeds, tahini.
DRINK distilled water, alfalfa tea, horsetail tea.

Pancreas Problems

The pancreas is a gland that is designed to produce enzymes. Some of the enzymes that are created here are used to digest proteins, fats and carbohydrates. Insulin for the metabolism of sugar is also manufactured here.

When problems begin in the pancreas they manifest in other functions of the body. Digestion is disrupted and constipation can also result. If the sugar in the blood that is used as fuel is not metabolized properly then you have an accumilation of that sugar. When the blood sugar stays at high levels, you have a disease called diabetes. (See Diabetes for more information).

It is obvious that it is important to nourish the pancreas and to keep it fit. Toning and nourishing the pancreas will prevent many distressing situations from taking place.

Here is a formula that is available in the marketplace today that would be beneficial for providing most of the nutritional support for this gland:

DANDELION ROOT	CEDAR BERRIES
GENTIAN ROOT	UVA URSI
ZINC	SELENIUM
MANGANESE	CYSTINE
LICORICE ROOT	ECHINACEA
WHEAT BRAN	SAFFLOWER FLOWERS
GOLDENSEAL ROOT	

Here are the nutrients and why they help:

HERBS

DANDELION ROOT: Stimulates bile production, benefit the spleen and improves the health of the pancreas.

GENTIAN ROOT: Its focus of activity is on those glands and organs involved in digestion, gallbladder and pancreas.

LICORICE ROOT: Strengthens the pancreas and spleen.

WHEAT BRAN: It lowers blood glucose levels and stimulates the pancreas to produce their own insulin. Enzymes active in the fundus of the stomach are preferred.

GOLDENSEAL ROOT: Lowers blood sugar and stimulates the pancreas.

CEDAR BERRIES: Stimulates the pancreas.

UVA URSI: As an astringent it is used as a tonic and specific in cases involving weakened liver, kidneys and other glands.

ECHINACEA: Is absorbed into the kidneys, cleanses and strenthens that organ, liver, spleen and pancreas.

SAFFLOWER FLOWERS: Encourages the pancreas to manufacture natural insulin.

MINERALS

ZINC: Plays a part in manufacturing of insulin in the pancreas.
MANGANESE: Stores of it are found chiefly in the human liver, kidney, pancreas, lungs, prostate gland, adrenals and brain.
SELENIUM: Is very good for the liver and pancreas.
CYSTINE: Supplies an appreciable amount of insulin needed by the pancreas for assimilation of sugars and starches.

Knowing that you can find these nutrients in a formula that will deliver most of the prime ingredients, here is how I recommend to take them: 1 or 2 capsules at each meal. If diabetes is present then you need to work with Program M-Dia as discussed in the Diabetes segment.

SPECIAL DIETARY CONSIDERATIONS

ELIMINATE fatty foods.

Parasites

Excellent for ridding the intestinal tract of PARASITES. The concept here is to kill the parasites on contact as well as deprive them of their food (blood supply).

There are many different schools of thought in relationship to parasites and the role that they play in creating disease. LaDean Griffin, noted healer and author, stated in a booklet that she felt parasites were a cause of diabetes.

Her theory is that they invade the pancreas and therefore interfere with its working. In this way the insulin producing capabilities of the pancreas are reduced and excessive sugar builds up in the blood stream.

Another healer feels that parasites are the cause of tumors and cysts. Others feel that parasites in the intestinal tract rob the body of needed nutrition and thus lower the health and vitality of the body. This sets in motion the receptivity for disease.

Regardless of which particular way that you may feel it is still prudent to eliminate parasites from the body. The easiest way to do it is with herbs.

Here is a formula that is available in the marketplace today that would be beneficial for providing most of the nutritional support for this condition:

Papaya Seeds	Garlic
Pumpkin Seeds	Wormseed
Black Walnut	Wood Betony
Pau D'Arco	Butternut Bark

Here is how these herbs work in the body:

PAPAYA SEEDS: Used extensively in Mexico as a way of ridding the body of parasites and worms.

PUMPKIN SEEDS: A non-irritating diuretic, its main use continues to be as an anthelmintic.

BLACK WALNUT: Used to expel various kinds of worms, high tannin content.

GARLIC: Increases resistance against bacterial infection and has been proven to have this effect on the following germs: Staphylococcus (Staph), Streptococcus (Strept), Vibrio Cholerae (Cholera), B. Typhosus (Typhus), B. Diphtheria (Diphtheria), B. Enteritides (Dysentery). Combats the following fungi: Candida albicans, Microsporum, Epidermophyton.

BUTTERNUT ROOT BARK: Most mild and efficacious laxatives known, not only as a laxative, but as a treatment for liver disorders (as practiced extensively in homeopathy) and intestinal sickness. It increased the manufacture and secretion of bile and increased the activity of glands in the walls of the intestinal tract.

PAU D'ARCO: Used in all situations that deal with bacteria. Fungus cannot grow around this tree.

WORMSEED: Also known as Jerusalem Artichoke. Known for its ability to kill parasites.

Knowing that you can find these nutrients in a formula that will deliver most of the prime ingredients, here is how I recommend to take them: 2 or 3 at each meal and 2 before bed.

SPECIAL DIETARY CONSIDERATIONS

INCREASE consumption of garlic, onions, celery and all the fresh vegetables and fruits possible. This will act as roughage and bulk material to push out the toxic parasites and fungus that will be killed by the herbs.

Pre Menstrual Syndrome

P.M.S. (pre menstrual syndrome) has generated a lot of interest over the past few years as medical and nutritional sciences acknowledge the fact that this condition does truly exist. For the most part it is largely ignored by the medical profession because they don't know what to do about it. Of course their normal approach is to give the woman a drug, generally a tranquilizer, to help her feel better. This is a standard medical approach to most physical conditions.

Fortunately there is another, more sensible, approach. One that is based on the knowledge that the human body is created out of nutrients, such as proteins, fats, carbohydrates and water. It also requires vitamins and minerals to function at optimum health. With this perception nutritional science looks at every disease and discomfort as the result of nutritional deficiencies.

Now in order to come up with a nutritional program that will work you need to go back and look at the symptoms of Pre Menstrual Syndrome.

The most common and basic signs are: fluid retention, painful breasts, feelings of bloated stomach, headaches, backaches, skin eruptions, mental depression, irritability and lethargy.

It is very interesting to note that many of these symptoms are the same for candida and that some women prior to their menstrual cycle have a discharge. This could this be from the fact that as the body prepares to cleanse it under goes a degree of stress and stress lowers the immune system, this allows the candida that has been held in check to flourish. This causing the P.M.S. to be experienced and viewed as a separate condition.

Let's take a look at how stress effects the body. Stress taxes the adrenal glands which secrete hormones that carry messages to the other glands on how and/or what to perform or manufacture. All of the glands of the body are tied together in a complicated system. Each and every aspect of life within the body is dependent on each other. This is why it is so important to maintain a proper nutritional balance within. In this way you are providing the system with the needed ingredients to function correctly and thus provide optimum health. It also eliminates the opportunity for disease to take hold.

Here is a formula that is available in the marketplace today that would be beneficial for providing most of the nutritional support for this condition:

GLA (gamma lanic acid)	Magnesium (amino acid chelate)
Vitamin B1	Iron (amino acid chelate)
Vitamin B6	Zinc (amino acid chelate)
Vitamin C	Licorice
Niacin (B3)	Corn Silk
Pantothenic Acid (B5)	Parsley
Calcium (amino acid chelate)	Watermelon Seed

Valerian Root
Wild Lettuce
Horsetail Grass
Suma

Blessed Thistle
Squaw Vine
False Unicorn Root
White Willow Bark

Here is how the nutrients work in the body:

VITAMINS

VITAMIN B1: Known as the "morale vitamin" to a healthy nervous system and its beneficial effect on mental attitude.
VITAMIN B6: Helps maintain the balance of sodium and potassium, which regulates body fluids and promotes the normal functioning of the nervous and musculoskeletal systems.
VITAMIN C: This nutrient, along with vitamin B6, B3 (niacin), and Zinc are vital co-factors in the production of additional GLA.
NIACIN (B3): GLA co-factor.
PANTOTHENIC ACID (B5): Nourishes the adrenal glands. Helps to provide energy.

MINERALS

CALCIUM: Acts as a calming agent and to relieve backaches.
MAGNESIUM: For the assimilation of calcium. To relax muscles and nerves.
IRON: Depletion can cause fatigue, inability to concentrate, paleness, and lack of muscle tone.
ZINC: Another co-factor for GLA.

HERBS

LICORICE: Estrogenic activity.
CORN SILK: Used extensively for the reduction of fluids.
PARSLEY: Excellent for reducing fluid retention.
WATERMELON SEED: Good for reducing fluids.
VALERIAN ROOT: Valerian root and / or its major constituents, the valepotriates, have marked sedative anticonvulsive, hypotensive, tranquilizing neurotropic, and anti-aggressive properties.
WILD LETTUCE: As a sedative on the central nervous system.
HORSETAIL GRASS: One of the best sources of silica which is essential for calcium assimilation and utilization. Silica also transmutes into calcium.
SUMA: Invigorates the female hormonal balance without disturbing effects.
BLESSED THISTLE: For headaches and any kind of female problem.
SQUAW VINE: Very good for the feelings of morning sickness or nausea. Also contains significant amounts of the amino acid tryptophan, known for its calming effects.

FALSE UNICORN ROOT: Great for all female problems. Helps in reducing headaches and depression.

OTHER SYNERGISTIC NUTRIENTS

GLA (gammalinolenic acid): Essential for the production of prostaglandins which are regulators for the cells. This helps to smooth out the rapidly changing hormone levels during the menstrual cycle.

Knowing that you can find these nutrients in a formula that will deliver most of the prime ingredients, here is how I recommend to take them: start off with 2 (two) tablets at breakfast and then 1 (one) or 2 (two) tablets at lunch. Wait to see how you feel if you need another tab or two that would be fine. Try not to take too many late in the day as you may find that you have too much energy, this may create a problem trying to go to sleep.

Every human body has a slightly different bio-chemical composition, therefore in some instances it becomes necessary to take more of a supplement than what is suggested.

SPECIAL DIETARY CONSIDERATIONS

INCREASE vitamin B6, 10 days preceding menstruation. Also helpful is vitamin B12 and Kelp is of specific importance and calming herbs such as alfalfa, hops and vitamin E.
DRINK hyssop tea and scullcap (mixed with Pennroyal) tea.

Prostate Problems

REDUCES PROSTATE INFLAMMATION, nourishes and strengthens prostate gland.

The prostate gland, like other glands, organs and systems in the body, is subject to certain physical problems.

It appears that many men over the age of 50 seem to suffer from an inflamed prostate gland. The inflammation is sometimes painful and almost always uncomfortable.

By eliminating whatever the physical causes, you may be able to increase the speed of healing. Another step would be to increase the use of those nutrients that are known to be beneficial to the prostate.

Here is a formula that is available in the marketplace today that would be beneficial for providing most of the nutritional support for this condition:

Vitamin E (D-Alpha Tocopheryl)	Glycine (Amino Acid)
Unsaturated Fatty Acids	Bee Pollen
Zinc (Amino Acid Chelate)	Parsley
Magnesium (Amino Acid Chelate)	Pumpkin Seed
Glutamic Acid (Amino Acid)	Echinacea
Alanine (Amino Acid)	Gravel Root

Here is how the nutrients work in the body:

VITAMINS

VITAMIN E & UNSATURATED FATTY ACIDS: Essential for glandular health and work together in lessening of residual urine.

AMINO ACIDS

GLUTAMIC ACID, ALANINE AND GLYCINE: These amino acids are important; their role in human nutrition is extensive and not completely known.

HERBS

POLLEN: Contains various nutrients that are strengthening and beneficial to the body.
PARSLEY & GRAVEL ROOT: Herbs known to reduce inflammation.
PUMPKIN SEEDS: High in zinc.

OTHER SYNERGISTIC NUTRIENTS

ZINC: An essential mineral for the normal functioning of the prostate gland.

Knowing that you can find these nutrients in a formula that will deliver most of the prime ingredients, here is how I recommend to take them: For severe inflammation: 1 tablet every hour for the first 2 days, then 1 each meal.

This combination could be taken frequently throughout the first couple of days, 1 every hour or so, when there is severe inflammation.

Once the inflammation is reduced, then this combination could be used as a maintenance program.

SPECIAL DIETARY CONSIDERATIONS

ELIMINATE all sweets.

INCREASE bee pollen, alfalfa sprouts, green leafy vegetables, pumpkin seeds, parsley, nopales (cactus), string beans, vegetable oil in salads.

DRINK sarsaparilla tea.

Stress and Tension
Hyperactivity

PROGRAM M-TRQ

Tranquilizer

A natural TRANQUILIZER that is effective for reducing and eliminating the dependence of pharmaceutical tranquilizers. Also useful as a SLEEPING formula, especially effective when used in combination with a multi-mineral. Excellent for HYPERACTIVE CHILDREN until dietary changes are instituted. Should not be used by parents in place of those changes.

It is often said that stress is a killer, both directly and indirectly. Stress is known to cause heart attacks, high blood pressure, strokes, depression and is a contributory factor to lowering the immune system.

To begin with, stress creates physical tension in the muscles. This in turn limits the amount of blood that can flow through the arteries, veins and capillaries that are located in that area. When the blood flow is reduced due to tension there can often times be pain or cramping in that area.

Heart attacks are a specific example of what happens when blood is reduced to an area. It is also true that some heart attacks are caused by elevated cholesterol levels. Another good example of stress and tension at work is the common headache and migraines. These are usually brought on by stress and once the muscles tense and blood flow is reduced the headache begins. Blood carries oxygen and other nutrients to nerves and muscles. When these become starved they begin to experience pain.

Stress lowers the immune system by adversely effecting the adrenal glands. Through affecting the adrenal glands many different diseases may flourish. The main reason being that the adrenals are tied into other glands and their functions by the hormones that are produced in the adrenals. Hypoglycemia is a non-bacterial type of disease that is partially created through exhausted adrenals. Bacterial type diseases are able to flourish because of how the adrenals are tied into the thymus gland which is the "center" of the immune system.

Depression on the other hand is not looked at from a physical point of view but more as a mental, emotional situation. Everything that is caused by emotions, whether it's depression or "stress" or anger or whatever, is the direct response of how we look at something and how we react to what we are seeing. Therefore all mental and emotional stress is caused by perception. In order to reduce stress from this point of view a deep questioning program would be necessary. If you desire to pursue this course of action, then write to me, Neil Kelly care of the publisher.

Some forms of stress are caused by the environment. This includes the air we breathe, water we drink, food we eat, places we work. Because of all these different sources of stress it is important to maintain an excellent diet and to fortify the body with those nutrients that will help the body deal with stress. A healthy and nutritionally sound body deals with the stresses of life from a position of strength. This means that although there is stress, the body is not adversely affected by it.

Unfortunately, the American diet is so nutritionally deficient that there aren't enough nutrients available to keep the body fit and able. Stress depletes such nutrients as Calcium, Vitamin C and the entire range of B vitamins. This depletion can cause feelings of nervousness, irritability, sleeplessness and even muscle cramping. There are other physical results as well. The best way to deal with these depletions is to provide the body with the nutrients necessary.

The following program works to NOURISH AND RELAX NERVES AND MUSCLES, INDUCES CALM. Prepares body for sleep / rest.

Here is a formula that is available in the marketplace today that would be beneficial for providing most of the nutritional support for this condition:

Calcium (Amino Acid Chelate)	Lady Slipper
Magnesium (Amino Acid Chelate)	Hops
L-Tryptophan (Amino Acid)	Inositol
L-Tyrosine (Amino Acid)	Vitamin B6 (Pyridoxine)
Valerian Root	Niacinamide
Scullcap	

Here is how the nutrients work in the body:

HERBS
VALERIAN, SKULLCAP, LADY SLIPPER AND HOPS: All used for ages to nourish, soothe and relax the nerves and muscles.

VITAMINS
VITAMIN B6: Essential for healthy nerve endings.
INOSITOL: Acts in a calming way on the nervous system.

OTHER SYNERGISTIC NUTRIENTS
L-TRYPTOPHAN: An amino acid known for its calming effect.
L-TYROSINE: An amino acid known to elevate moods.
CALCIUM AND MAGNESIUM: Work to nourish and relax nerves and muscles.

Knowing that you can find these nutrients in a formula that will deliver most of the prime ingredients, here is how I recommend to take them: For anxiety — 1 every hour until calm restored. For insomnia — 3 or 4 tablets a 1 / 2 hour before bed for first 3 nights, then 1 or 2 before bed.

SPECIAL DIETARY CONSIDERATIONS
ELIMINATE caffeine, artificial flavors, colors and flavors, sweets.
INCREASE dark, leafy greens, sesame seeds or tahini.
DRINK skullcap tea, chamomile tea, peppermint tea.

Thymus Problems

The thymus gland is involved with the immune system in many important ways. It is rare that there are physical problems with this gland. To be on the safe side, especially with the threat of AIDS in the world it may pay to insure that this gland stays in top shape.

So with that in mind I have found a formula that does just that.

Here is the formula that is available in the marketplace today that would be beneficial for providing most of the nutritional support for this gland:

L-ARGININE   LECITHIN
L-GLYCINE   BETA CAROTENE
ZINC

Here are the nutrients and why they help:

MINERALS

L-ARGININE: Growth hormone acts on the thymus gland to improve its ability to process T-effector and B-cell lymphocytes.

L-GLYCINE: Necessary for the immune system, for balanced growth of white blood cells and for health of the thymus gland, spleen and bone marrow.

ZINC: Protects the immune system and supports the T-cells.

LECITHIN: Increases resistance to disease by helping the thymus gland carry out its functions.

BETA CAROTENE: Is converted into Vitamin A in the body. As Vitamin A it feeds and strengthens the thymus gland, which is responsible for how the body responds to infections.

Knowing that you can find these nutrients in a formula that will deliver most of the prime ingredients, here is how I recommend to take them: 1 or 2 at each meal.

Thyroid Problems

The thyroid is a very important gland because of its interactions with other glands. In fact the thyroid is often called the "master gland or power control center".

It secretes two hormones having a specific iodine requirement and which vitality influence the rate and processes of basic body metabolism and physical growth.

Goiter is the result of hyper-activity within the thyroid.

Here is a formula that is available in the marketplace today that would be beneficial for providing most of the nutritional support for this gland:

GTF CHROMIUM
TYROSINE
KELP
MANGANESE

BLADDERWRACK
GENTIAN
VITAMIN B6
IRISH MOSS

Here are the nutrients and why they help:

HERBS

BLADDERWRACK: Has been effective against thyroid problems.
IRISH MOSS: Provides iodine, and is a form of kelp.

MINERALS

GTF CHROMIUM: Can stimulate thyroid activity to initiate the mobilization of fat reserves for energy production.
TYROSINE: Plays an integral role in proper functioning of the adrenal, pituitary and thyroid gland.
KELP: Kelp and the Mosses, thyroid, parathyroid, pineal and pituitary, need in order to adequately function well.
MANGANESE: Is essential for the formation of thyroxin, a constituent of the thyroid gland.
GENTIAN: Bitter principles that are known to normalize the functioning of the thyroid, through an indirect means.

VITAMINS

VITAMIN B6: Involved in nourishing the adrenal glands, reduces water content and inflammation. Excellent in metabolizing fats, proteins and carbohydrates.

Knowing that you can find these nutrients in a formula that will deliver most of the prime ingredients, here is how I recommend to take them: 1 or 2 at each meal.

SPECIAL DIETARY CONSIDERATIONS

INCREASE carrot-celery-parsley and spinach juice, vitamins C and E and olive oil. Among the vegetables containing the best supply of vitamin C and E are spinach, lettuce, and watercress together with carrots and green peppers.

DRINK parsley juice mixed with carrot, celery, lettuce or spinach.

Ulcer Problems

Everyone is well aware of what causes ulcers, so let's look at some very simple but highly effective "cures".

The most effective and quickest is:

One (1) teaspoon of cayenne powder mixed into a cup of hot water. Let stand to "room tempature" and drink immediately before going to bed.

By the next morning there will no longer be an ulcer to bother you. This treatment seems to last for years.

Two other approaches, and not as "tasty" are:

Drink one ounce of aloe vera juice as frequently as possible. Or drink fresh made cabbage juice as often as possible. Keep in mind the potential for intestinal gases.

Last but not least is a chewable wafer that offers relief without all the "tasty alternatives". This wafer is slightly sweetened with herbs.

Here is a formula that is available in the marketplace today that would be beneficial for providing most of the nutritional support for this condition:

SLIPPERY ELM	WILD CHERRY BARK
LICORICE	OKRA
MARSHMALLOW	SWEET LEAF
CABBAGE JUICE	

Here are the nutrients and why they help:

HERBS

SLIPPERY ELM: Internally soothes irritated mucous membranes. Very valuable for mucous inflammation of the stomach. Will sustain ulcerated and cancerous stomach.

LICORICE: Relieves ulcer conditions, also used for flavor.

MARSHMALLOW: It soothes mucous membranes. Internally to treat inflammation and mucosal afflictions of the genito-urinary tract.

CABBAGE JUICE: A natural antiseptic used to ease ulcer pain; heals ulcers.

WILD CHERRY BARK: Used for flavor.

SWEET LEAF: Used for flavor.

Knowing that you can find these nutrients in a formula that will deliver most of the prime ingredients, here is how I recommend to take them: chew 1 or 2 wafers as needed.

SPECIAL DIETARY CONSIDERATIONS

ELIMINATE anything that can irritate the mucous membranes of the stomach and duodenum from the diet. This includes whole grains, nuts and whole-grain bread and cereals. Avoid raw fruits, vegetables, sour fruits, and fried foods. Strictly avoided: tobacco, alcohol, coffee, tea, chocolate, salt and strong spices such as white and black pepper, mustard, vinegar, chili, etc. Also white sugar, soft drinks, drinks that are too hot or too cold.

INCREASE frequent small meals. Potatoes, squash, yams, avocados, and raw bananas. Well cooked millet cereal with milk, cooked white rice with milk. Include complete relaxation and avoidance of all mental stress and worries.

DRINK raw cabbage and potato juice; vitamins E and A, comfrey tea; goat's milk; brewer's yeast. Also included is carrot, beet, and cucumber juice. Water may also ease the pain.

Vision Problems

See CATARACTS, GLAUCOMA : PROGRAM M-VI

Water Retention

PROGRAM M-WA

A natural well balanced DIURETIC.

This particular program is designed to equalize water pressure on a cellular level.

Here is a formula that is available in the marketplace today that would be beneficial for providing most of the nutritional support for this condition:

Vitamin B6 (Pyridoxine)
Potassium (Amino Acid Chelate)
Corn Silk
Buchu
Uva-Ursi

Hydrangea
Elder Flowers
Parsley
Watermelon Seed
Samphire

Here is how these nutrients work in the body:

HERBS

CORN SILK, BUCHU, UVA URSI, HYDRANGEA, PARSLEY, WATERMELON: all are excellent diuretics.

OTHER SYNERGISTIC NUTRIENTS

POTASSIUM, VITAMIN B6: Work together to maintain the fluid balance of the body.

Knowing that you can find these nutrients in a formula that will deliver most of the prime ingredients, here is how I recommend to take them: 1 (one) or 2 two) at each meal.

SPECIAL DIETARY CONSIDERATIONS

ELIMINATE salt.

INCREASE the consumption of watermelon, pineapple, cucumber, parsley.

DRINK parsley tea, watermelon seed tea.

Weight Loss

Traditionally there are three basic approaches to diet and weight loss when using natural supplements. The use of diuretic type herbs to reduce water content. Intake of the lipo-tropic vitamins, better known as "fat burners", to reduce fat and cholesterol deposits. And the use of natural appetite suppressants to curb the craving for food.

These approaches are effective and each in its own right works, and works well. There are two major drawbacks with this type of approach. If you really want your weight loss program to be quick and highly effective then you are going to have to buy all the different items, the herbs, vitamins and appetite suppressants. The expense of buying all those different nutrients can create a meaningful dent in your bank account. Not to mention the inconvenience of taking any where from two to three tablets from each bottle. This just might add up to over 10 or 15 tablets each meal.

Now there is a better, much less expensive and more convenient method of accomplishing the same goals;

SYNERGISTICALLY COMPLETE NUTRITIONAL PROGRAMS IN A BOTTLE.

In essence a SYNERGISTIC approach incorporates all three categories of nutrient supplementation: diuretics, "fat burners" and appetite suppressants.

The following program BURNS FAT AWAY through lipotropic nutrients, INCREASES BASIC METABOLISM, FLUSHES OUT EXCESS FLUIDS.

Here is a formula that is available in the marketplace today that would be beneficial for providing most of the nutritional support for this condition:

> Lecithin
> Choline (Bitartrate)
> Inositol
> L-Methionine (Free Form Amino Acid)
> L-Phenylalanine (Free Form Amino Acid)
> Vitamin B6 (Pyridoxine)
> Potassium (Amino Acid Complex)
> Kelp
> Chickweed
> Seawrack
> White Ash

Here is how the nutrients work in the body:

VITAMINS

LECITHIN, CHOLINE, INOSITOL: Often used to reduce the fatty deposits within the body by dissolving them. Lecithin acts as a carrier of fat molecules and pulls them out of the body. **VITAMIN B6:** Acts as a diuretic.

HERBS

SEAWRACK AND WHITE ASH: Act as diuretics in the body.

OTHER SYNERGISTIC NUTRIENTS

METHIONINE: An amino acid that aids the body in producing Choline.
PHENYLALANINE: Another amino acid. This one is converted to Norepinephrine in the body, which reduces hunger.
POTASSIUM: Acts as a diuretic by balancing fluids.
KELP: Contains iodine which nourishes the thyroid gland and helps to regulate metabolism.

Knowing that you can find these nutrients in a formula that will deliver most of the prime ingredients, here is how I recommend to take them: 1 or 2 tablets each meal.

SPECIAL DIETARY CONSIDERATIONS

ELIMINATE all sugar, salt, white flour products, starchy foods, sodas, cut down on meat, chicken and fish, no fried foods.
INCREASE vegetables — all raw and fresh, cucumbers, parsley, carrots, cauliflower, garlic. Fruits — bananas, watermelon, cherries, grapes, figs, prunes, pineapple, 1 / 2 grapefruit before each meal, 1 / 2 fresh squeezed lemon juice in the morning on an empty stomach.
DRINK corn silk tea, watermelon seed tea, or buchu or uva ursi teas. Another thing that can be done when you stop losing weight and can't seem to lose any more is to "break the magic line" with 10 fresh squezzed lemons into two (2) quarts of distilled water and drink over a two (2) day period. This drink acts as a super liver cleansor and it speeds up the body's ability to digest "fat".

Salves and
Lotions

Acne and
Skin Problems

FORMULATION M-DER / 1

Good as a topical dressing in all skin problems, especially ACNE, ECZEMA, PSORIASIS, FUNGUS under the nails and in the scalp.

To speed up the external beautification process, a topical dressing of herbs would be helpful. A good way to apply such herbs would be in an oil base. In this way, you topically feed the skin what it needs and at the same time the herbal properties are working their magic.

The following herbs, in oil form, will act as ANTIFUNGAL, ANTIVIRAL, and ASTRINGENT agents.

Here is a list of herbal oils and what those herbal oils do on the skin:

GOLDENSEAL ROOT, PAU D'ARCO, AND BLACK WALNUT: Have all been used to kill bacteria.
LEMON PEEL, WITCH HAZEL, AND QUEEN OF THE MEADOW: Are astringent herbs used to tighten pores.
ECHINACEA: Also has anti-septic properties.
CALENDULA AND COMFREY: Are famous for the healing properties on the skin.

This combination can also be used for athlete's foot, fungus under the nails and "sores" in the scalp.

Apply as needed to face, body, scalp, nails.

Burns

(All Types)

Instant relief from SUNBURN. Great also for all OTHER TYPES OF BURNS. Makes a good MASSAGE OIL.

Even with the best suntan lotions, your skin can be, and often is, burnt, dried and chapped after a day in the summer sun. Every time the skin is exposed and burnt by the sun it becomes etched with tiny "aging" lines. Your face is the first area to show these lines because of the extensive exposure to the sun and elements. Together they damage cells that will age and wrinkle your skin.

There are certain oils and special herbs that can counteract some of the harsh damage, and at the same time, cool down and soothe the skin.

The following is such a cooling and soothing combination. It is ideal for the immediate relief from the discomfort of too much sun.

Here is a list of the herbal oils and what they do for the skin:

WHITE CAMPHOR OIL: Cools down the skin on contact.

CALENDULA, COMFREY, MARSHMALLOW, CHAMOMILE AND SLIPPERY ELM: Excellent for soothing and nourishing the skin. Each herb has certain qualities that work on as well as beneath the skin. In oil form, their special properties penetrate and nourish the skin at cellular levels.

VITAMINS A AND E: Used extensively for the healing and repairing of damaged skin.

ALMOND OIL: Probably the most effective beauty oil in the world today. It quickly penetrates, nourishes and softens the skin on contact.

This combination is also great for use as an after bath oil or even during the bath for a nourishing and soothing soak, and a fantastic massage oil too.

Chest Rub

FORMULATION M-VA/s

Good for all types of LUNG CONGESTION. Works like Vicks Vapo Rub, only stronger and 100% natural.

The following herbs should be used in salve form for the best results:

OILS OF EUCALYPTUS, WINTERGREEN, PEPPERMINT.
GARLIC may also be added as a topical anti-biotic that will travel into the lungs.

Apply as needed.

Ear Infections

FORMULATION M-G/1

Excellent for EAR INFECTIONS. Also good for loosening hard ear wax. The following herbs in oil form would be the best way to get results:

GARLIC AND GOLDENSEAL ROOT because of their ability to kill bacteria.

Apply 2-4 drops in affected ear 4 times per day.

Headaches

FORMULATION M-WP/s

The following oils should be used in a salve form for the best results:

OILS OF PEPPERMINT AND WINTERGREEN.

Apply as frequently as possible or needed.

Hemorrhoids

FORMULATION M-RE/s

Formulated to reduce HEMORRHOIDS. Works like Preparation H, only better and stronger. Also good for varicose veins. Has been used for puffiness under eyes, however essential oils will sting the eyes, Astringent, anti-inflammatory, pain reliever.

The following herbs should be used in salve form for best results.

BAYBERRY, WHITE OAK, GOLDENSEAL ROOT, MYRRH.

Apply as needed 3-4 times per day.

Joint Problems (Pain)
FORMULATION M-PA/s

Natural PAIN relief for all types of pain. Works like Ben Gay, only stronger and 100 % natural.

For muscle and joint pain apply to muscles and joints as needed. For head pain apply as needed — rub over the sinuses, into the temples and across the nape of the neck.

OIL OF WINTERGREEN should be made into a salve.

Psoriasis and Planter Warts
FORMULATION M-PS/s

A specific salve prepared for PSORIASIS. Also proven effective against planter's warts and other hard to eliminate skin viruses.

I believe that Psoriasis is a bacterial condition which is caused by a traumatic event in a person's life. That event stresses the body to such a point that the immune system ceases to function. During that period of "no protection" a virus takes hold and builds a home.

Now it is a proven fact that stress does lower the body's immune system. Research is continuing in that area because of the implication that stress may be a contributing factor in some diseases.

If we continue to follow the thought that Psoriasis may well be a viral type infection, then we need to deal with it from that point of view. To do so, a topical dressing would work directly against such a virus is needed.

The following herbs should be in salve form for best results:

OILS OF PEPPERMINT AND LEMONGRASS: Have been used to treat viral conditions.
GOLDENSEAL ROOT, MYRRH, CHICKWEED AND PAU D'ARCO: Have been employed for hundreds of years for their antifungal properties.
COMFREY: Excellent for tissue rebuilding and cellular health.

This type of combination can be applied as frequently as desired or needed.

It should be noted that if the skin is "open" from whatever the problem, the Oils of Peppermint and Lemongrass may sting.

This feeling will usually disappear within 10-20 minutes.

Sinus Decongestant
FORMULATION M-SI / 1

This combination of herbs in tincture form will FIGHT BACTERIA, BREAK UP SINUS CONGESTION, and REDUCE INFLAMMATION.

GOLDENSEAL ROOT, ECHINACEA, BAYBERRY, WHITE OAK.

Apply as needed.

Skin Problem (Itching)
FORMULATION M-IT / s

Natural itch relief. May also be effective in killing low grade skin infections.

These herbs should be made into a salve for best results:

GOLDENSEAL ROOT, WINTERGREEN AND CLOVE OIL.

Apply as needed.

Vaginitis (Yeast Infections)
FORMULATION M-FE / P / 1

A strong DOUCHE designed to eliminate yeast infections rapidly. An excellent combination of tinctured herbs is:

GOLDENSEAL ROOT: The most widely used anti-biotic herb employed by herbalists. It is highly effective both internally, in caps, tablets and teas; and externally, as a wash and douche.

PAU D'ARCO: Became an important herb in the anti-fungal arsenal since its reported use against cancer. It is true that fungus will not grow on the bark of this tree.

BLACK WALNUT: Another herb used in dealing with fungi, parasites, intestinal worms and other foreign invaders. Some herbalists use it to combat tumors.

THYME AND MYRRH: Have anti-septic properties. The germicidal properties of Myrrh also increase the white blood cell count when taken internally.

Knowing that you can find this herbal tincture in a formula that will deliver the prime ingredients, here is how I recommend to work with it: as a douche, use it 3 to 4 times in succession, i.e. upon awakening, midday if possible or immediately after work, before bed, and again at wake-up.

Warts and
Low Grade Fungus

FORMULATION M-VR/s

The following herbs should be used in salve form for best results:

GOLDENSEAL ROOT, MYRRH, OILS OF PEPPERMINT AND LEMONGRASS: All have the ability to kill skin bacteria.

Apply as frequently as possible.

Food Notes

The following foods, once consumed, will increase the ACID content of the blood. Therefore the amounts consumed should be kept to a minimum: MOST MEATS, FISH, FOWL, and GRAINS, WHOLE WHEAT PRODUCTS, NUTS (EXCEPT BRAZIL AND ALMONDS), DAIRY AND LEGUMES.

The following foods are ALKALIZING FOODS: Figs, soybean, lima beans, apricots, spinach, turnip, beet tops, raisins, millet, buckwheat, sprouts, vegetable and fruit juices, vegetable broth.

Minerals In Foods

CALCIUM

Almonds, carrots, dandelions, turnips, spinach, oranges, goat's milk, okra, cauliflower, tomatoes, garlic, berries, nuts, apples, potatoes, apricots, comfrey, horsetail grass.

PHOSPHOROUS

Kale, parsley, radish (white), asparagus, watercress, brussels sprouts, garlic, carrots, cauliflower, squash, cucumbers, lettuce, turnips, mission figs, oranges, limes, cherries, blackberries, brazil nuts, walnuts.

POTASSIUM

Carrots, celery, parsley, spinach, beets, cauliflower, garlic, raw potato, squash, tomatoes, turnips, oranges, lemons, apricots, banana, cherries, dates, grapes, figs, pears, peaches, plums, watermelon, olives. Brussels sprouts, kale, horseradish, cauliflower, cabbage, chives, garlic, cranberries, raspberries, pineapple, currants, apples, brazil nuts, filberts.

MAGNESIUM

Carrots, celery, cucumbers, almonds, dandelion, garlic, kale, lettuce, tomatoes, spinach, lemons, oranges, apples, bananas, figs, pineapple, brazil nuts, pecans, pinons, walnuts.

IRON

Lettuce, carrots, dandelion, radish, asparagus, turnips, cucumbers, horseradish, tomatoes, almonds, avocado, figs, strawberries, raisins, figs, watermelon, apricots, plums, beets, cherries, walnuts, brazil nuts, apples, concord grapes, pineapple.

MANGANESE

Parsley, carrots, celery, beets, cukes, almonds, apples, apricots, walnuts, buckwheat, peas, beans, nuts.

Bibliography and Suggested Reading

DISEASES

A BAREFOOT DOCTOR'S MANUAL, Victor W. Sidell, M.D.

ALL FALL DOWN, (Aids and the End of Circulation), William Campbell Douglass, M.D.

AMERICAN FOLK MEDICINE, Clarence Meyer

THE BEST OF LINDA CLARK, Some Unusual Approaches to Health, Linda Clark, M.A.

BIOCHEMICAL INDIVIDUALITY, Roger J. Williams

CANDIDA ALBICANS, Ray C. Wunderlich, Jr., M.D. and Dwight K. Kalita, Ph.D.

CANCER, Causes, Prevention and Treatment, The Total Approach, Paa vo Airola, Ph.D., N.D.

CATARACTS, Kurt W. Donsbach, Ph.D., D.Sc., N.D., D.C. and Dr. Alex Duarte, Optometrist

ENZYME NUTRITION, Dr. Edward Howell

FOLK MEDICINE, D.C. Jarvies, M.D.

HEALING AIDS NATURALLY, Laurence E. Badgley, M.D.

HERPES! Something Can Be Done About It, Nicholas Sampsidis, M.S.

HOW TO GET WELL, Paavo Airola, N.D., Ph.D.

IMMUNOLOGY, AGING, and CANCER, F.M. Burnet

KNOW YOUR NUTRITION, Linda Clark, M.A.

LET'S GET WELL, Adelle Davis

MUSCULESS DIET HEALING SYSTEM, Prof. Arnold Ehret

NUTRITIONAL GUIDE for the PREVENTION and CURE of COMMON AILMENTS and DISEASES, Carlton Fredericks, Ph.D.

OUR EARTH OUR CURE, Raymond Dextreit

SCLEROLOGY, Kurt W. Donsbach, Ph.D., N.D., D.C.

WELLNESS WORKBOOK, Regina Sara Ryan and John W. Travis, M.D.

YOU DON'T HAVE TO DIE, Harry S. Hoxsey, N.D.

YOUR HEARTS DESIRE, GOOD HEALTH, Calvin G. Dence, N.D.

ZEN MACROBIOTICS, Georges Ohsawa

FOODS

APPLE CIDER VINEGAR SYSTEM, Paul C. Bragg, N.D. Ph.D., Patricia Bragg, Ph.D.

BOOK OF SALADS, Joan Lay, N.D., M.B.N.O.A.

THE COMPLETE BOOK OF SPICES, John Heinerman

FOOD ITS INFLUENCE AS A FACTOR IN DISEASE and HEALTH, J.H. Tilden, M.D.

FRESH VEGETABLE and FRUIT JUICES, N.W. Walker, D.Sc.

HEINERMAN'S ENCYCLOPEDIA OF FRUITS, VEGETABLES and HERBS, John Heinerman

HERBAL COMBINATIONS from Authoritive Sources, Long Life Books

HERBAL CURES of DUODENAL ULCERS and GALL STONES, Frank Roberts

HERBAL HANDBOOK, Dawn McCleod

HERBAL HEALTH GUIDE, Neva Jensen

HERBAL RECIPES, David C. Meyer, Meyerbooks

HERBS TO THE RESCUE, LaDean Griffin

HERBS TO THE RESCUE II, LaDean Griffin

HOW INDIANS USE WILD PLANTS for FOOD, MEDICINES, and CRAFTS, Frances Densmore

INDIAN USES OF NATIVE PLANTS, Edith Van Allen Murphey

INSULIN vs HERBS and the DIABETIC, LaDean Griffin

NEW HOPE REAL HELP for those who have MULTIPLE SCLEROSIS, John Pageler

REGENERATING YOUR IMMUNE SYSTEM with FOODS and HERBS, John Heinerman

SEX DRUGS and APHRODISIACS, Adam Gottlieb

HERBS

BACK TO EDEN, Jethro Kloss

CHINESE HERBAL MEDICINE, Daniel P. Reid

CHINESE MEDICINAL HERBS, Compiled by, Li Shih-Chen, Translated and researched by F. Porter Smith, M.D. and G.A. Stuart, M.D.

COMPLETE HERBAL and ENGLISH PHYSICIAN, Mr. Nicholas Culpeper and Peter Cole

THE DICTIONARY OF MODERN HERBALISM, Simon Y. Mills, M.A. M.N.I.M.H.

ENCYCLOPEDIA DE PLANTAS MEDICINALES MEXICANAS, Heriberto Garcia Rivas

EVENING PRIMOSE OIL, Judy Graham

50 YEARS of THE HERBALIST ALMANAC, Clarence Meyer

HEALING ANIMALS WITH HERBS, John Heinerman

HERBAL AID, Edward Milo Millet

HERBAL DYNAMICS, John Heinerman

THE HERBALIST, Joseph E. Meyer, Revised and enlarged by Clarence Meyer

HERBAL RESEARCH MANUAL for PROFESSIONAL THERAPEUTICS, Compiled by John Heinerman

INDIAN HERBALOGY of NORTH AMERICA, Alma R. Hutchens

THE LITTLE HERB ENCYCLOPEDIA REVISED, Jack Ritchason

MAGIC HERBS for ARTHRITIS, RHEUMATISM, and related ailments, Richard Lucas

THE MAGICAL and RITUAL of HERBS, Richard Alan Miller

MEDICAL DOCTOR'S GUIDE TO HERBS, John Heinerman

THE PEOPLE'S HERBAL, Dr. Michael A. Weiner

PROVEN HERBAL REMEDIES, John H. Tobe

SCIENCE of HERBAL MEDICINE, John Heinerman

THE SCIENTIFIC VALIDATION of HERBAL MEDICINE, Daniel B. Mowrey, Ph.D.

SINGLE HERB LEAFLET, The Herbalist Magazine, Compiled by Health Ministry

TODAY'S HERBAL HEALTH, Louise Tenney

THE TREATMENT OF CANCER WITH HERBS, John Heinerman

THE WAY of HERBS, Michael Tierra, C.A.N.D.

VITAMINS and MINERALS

BODY, MIND, and the B VITAMINS, Ruth Adams and Frank Murray

THE BOOK OF VITAMIN THERAPY, Dr. Harold Rosenberg and A.N. Feldzamen, Ph.D.

CHOLINE, LECITHIN, INOSITOL and other Accessory Nutrients, Jeffrey Bland, Ph.D.

COMMON HERBS FOR NATURAL HEALTH, Juliette de Bairacli Levy

THE DICTIONARY OF VITAMINS, Leonard Mervyn B. Sc., Ph.D. C. Chem, F.R.S.C.

MINERALS: KILL OR CURE?, Ruth Adams and Frank Murray

NUTRITION ALAMANAC, Nutrition Search, Inc. John D. Kirschmann, Director, with Lavon J. Dunne

VITAMIN BIBLE, Earl Mindell

VITAMINS, MINERALS and NUTRITION, Elizabeth Somer, MA, RD

MISCELLANEOUS

A CONSUMER'S DICTIONARY of FOOD ADDITIVES, Ruth Winter

ACID and ALKALINE, Herman Aihara

AMINO ACIDS BOOK, Carlson Wade

AMINO ACIDS IN THERAPY, Leon Chaitow

THE ANATOMY COLORING BOOK, Wynn Kapit, Laurence M. Elson

THE BIOCHEMIC HANDBOOK, Formur, Inc. Publishers

CATALYST ALDRED WATER, Subcommittee on Health and Long-Term Care of the Select Committee on Aging US House of Representatives, Ninety-Sixth Congress

CHLORELLA, William H. Lee, R.Ph., Ph.D and Michael Rosenbaum, M.D.

DIGESTIVE ENZYMES, Jeffrey Bland, Ph.D.

HEALTH PLANTS of the WORLD, Francisco Bianchini, Francisco Corbetta, Marilena Pistoria

HOW TO USE THE 12 TISSUE SALTS, Esther Chapman

LIFE of the AZTECS in ANCIENT MEXICO, Pierre et Janine Soisson, translated by David Macrae

MIRACLE PROTEIN, Carlson Wade